# ALTERNATIVE MEDICINE
# OR
# MAGICAL HEALING

*"The trick is to know the difference."*

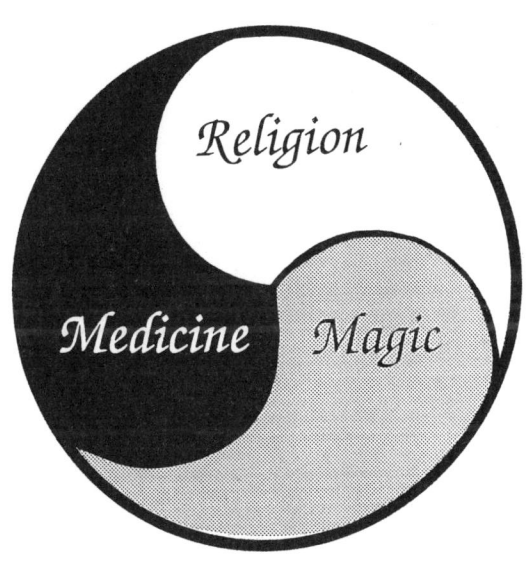

# ALTERNATIVE MEDICINE
# OR
# MAGICAL HEALING

*By*
**GEORGE A. ULETT, M.D., Ph.D.**

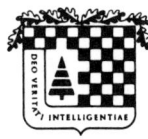

**WARREN H. GREEN, INC.**
St. Louis, Missouri, U.S.A.

*Published by*

WARREN H. GREEN, INC.
8356 Olive Boulevard
Saint Louis, Missouri 63132 U.S.A.

All rights reserved

© 1996 by WARREN H. GREEN, INC.

Second Printing, 1997

*Printed in the United States of America*

# ACKNOWLEDGMENTS

WITH THANKS to my wife Pearl, who was my companion in exploration of the lore of the Orient and the healing ways of the East. To Esther Schulz, Gretchen Smith, and Alisa Mixon for editorial and computer work on the manuscript, and Anne Barresi for her excellent editorial assistance at my publisher's, Warren H. Green, Inc. To Professor Ji Sheng Han for breakthroughs in neuroscience that led to scientized acupuncture. To neuroscientist Song Ping Han for aid and encouragement. To Mary Johnson and associates at the Missouri Institute of Mental Health Library for invaluable resource assistance. To Dr. Charles Cushing of the Christian Chiropractic Clinic in Asheville, North Carolina for guidance towards another way of looking at healing. My appreciation to the Ralph L. Smith Foundation for assistance in developing lecture material on Alternative Medicine for an enthusiastic audience, the medical students of Saint Louis University School of Medicine.

# PREFACE

THIS MANUAL about **alternative medicine** aims to explore that vast, ancient, often mystical, and relatively undisciplined mass of healing effort. Too many books on the subject are overly prejudiced — either enthusiastically for or vehemently against — the various topics that come under the umbrella of unconventional medicine. It is therefore important to present as unbiased a view as possible of what is in this vast storehouse of ideas from ancient traditions.

We have come a long way in the last 100 years in developing a system of medicine based on scientific evidence of effectiveness. Life expectancy has doubled, smallpox has been effectively eradicated, and many of the bacterial plagues that decimated populations in preceding centuries have been conquered. Before Pasteur's discovery of bacteria, four out of five children never reached adulthood. We can now treat acute infections and pneumonia, relieve much suffering, cure some cancers, and do other things previously thought to be impossible.

Why, then, do one third of all patients turn from modern scientific medicine to seek care at the hands of purveyors of alternative medicine with their ancient methods, often discarded or based on mysterious, metaphysical, unscientific, and unproven theories? The history of medicine is replete with quackery. Some people with no medical training, unable or unwilling to undergo the rigors of a scientific medical school education, find that unconventional healing techniques can present an easy way to "play doctor."

But medical quacks are not always deliberate frauds. Some simply lack the knowledge and training to distinguish between what is scientific and factual and what is baseless and false. Some persons are drawn to the mysterious, seeking some magic cure for their chronic patients. Many holistic healers cannot be dissuaded from a religious-like fascination with their erroneous beliefs. Finding like-minded companions, they form groups and revel together in the fantasy world of metaphysics.

In this manual, we will examine in an unbiased way what is offered by our friends in chiropractic, naturopathy, homeopathy, and acupuncture. They, too, are worshippers at the temple of Aesculapius. They are, in their own ways, reaching out to persons who are ill and hurting. Their motive, too, is to heal in whatever way they believe is correct. If there is something of value in their methods, let's find it.

My training as a physician would be considered orthodox by AMA standards. However, in my practice, I have often helped my patients by using such unconventional methods as hypnosis, testing for food allergies, suggestions for diet and exercise, megavitamin therapy, imagery, relaxation techniques, and acupuncture. As a psychiatrist, I am no stranger to mind/body medicine. Indeed, my practice is named *Psychosomatic Medicine and Psychiatry*.

Two decades ago, I became interested in Chinese acupuncture. Although I was fascinated, and for several years studied and practiced according to the cosmological beliefs and rules of this ancient healing profession, it became increasingly clear to me that if acupuncture worked, it must do so by some neurophysiological or biochemical means. I traveled to China, Japan, Hong Kong, Taiwan, and Scandanavia in search of facts. I found them, and as a result, was able to publish a small book entitled *Beyond Yin* and *Yang: How Acupuncture Really Works*. This became my text for teaching acupuncture to medical students. I find that students are eager to learn these alternative methods to supplement what they are learning about conventional medicine. After one of my lectures, a junior medical student said, "I plan to be an orthopedic surgeon, but if I can learn to use acupuncture, perhaps I can save some of my patients from unnecessary surgery." This would be preventive medicine at its best. And that is perhaps the greatest benefit to be found in the methods of alternative health care.

Giving attention to the whole person, mind and body, is a basic approach that characterizes such major alternative medical systems as Ayurvedic and Traditional Chinese Medicine. Beneath the layers of magic, mysticism, and strong placebo rituals, such systems emphasize the importance of examining the social factors, religion, and culture which form the patient's belief system. Practitioners of such systems of healing may also pay homage to preventive medicine by teaching their patients about proper diet, vitamins, minerals, exercise, and relaxation. Patients treated by alternative practitioners come away feeling that they have at last encountered a "caring physician" who listens, lays on hands, and gives emotional support.

Alternative medicine also defines a role for allied health professionals. Physicians' assistants, nurses, psychologists, physical therapists, dieticians, pharmacists, and others can all become members of the preventive health team using those techniques of alternative medicine that have been rigorously tested and have proven healing abilities. Added to medical practice, a renewed emphasis on preventive methods can be of great value. It is, however, unfortunate that what could clearly become a valuable adjunctive combination of alternative and allopathic methods has been sullied by opportunistic charlatans. Thus, one cannot embrace alternative medicine in its totality but rather must examine each proposed unconventional treatment in order to carefully sift the wheat from the chaff.

George Ulett, M.D., Ph.D.
St. Louis, Missouri
January 10, 1996

# TABLE OF CONTENTS

Preface .................................................................. vii

Introduction .......................................................... xiii

I. The Roots of Alternative Medicine – East and West ...... 3

II. Human Propensity for Magic and Mystery ................ 20

III. Placebo — The Power of "I Believe" ........................ 50

IV. Faith Healing ...................................................... 60

V. The Many Faces of Relaxation ............................... 79

VI. Holistic Hokum and Doubtful Diagnostic Procedures ....................................... 98

VII. Comprehensive Systems and Sideshows of Unconventional Medicine ............................ 116

VIII. Herbs and Homeopathy ..................................... 155

IX. Diet and Vitamins ............................................. 182

X. Acupuncture .................................................... 196

XI. Conclusion ...................................................... 218

Name Index ..................................................... 223

Subject Index .................................................. 229

# INTRODUCTION

A RECENT PAPER by Eisenberg (1) points out that as many as one in three Americans have used alternative methods of treatment. Currently, with the intensified focus on rising medical costs, all types of treatment have become topics of increased interest. Thus, unconventional methods have recently received much attention in the media. Books on the subject describing their assumed merits are found in all libraries and bookstores. Recently, the shelf space for such books has dramatically increased. Unfortunately however, these books for the most part have remained uncritically descriptive. Little attempt has been made to scientifically evaluate these treatments, to compare one with another, or to assess their worth in the manner of the scientific methods that are usually applied to allopathic medical techniques.

In 1992, the United States Congress appropriated two million dollars for the National Institutes of Health to establish an Office of Alternative Medicine. The director of this office, Joseph Jacobs, M.D., was a highly respected pediatrician and a Mohawk Indian, personally familiar with traditional healing methods. The office called for applications for research grants and received over 500 proposals. Funding permitted only 30 grants of $30,000 each, not nearly enough for any definitive studies. Dr. Jacobs resigned in September, 1994, and expressed frustration over militant purveyors of alternative therapies who were reluctant to submit their methods to careful scientific clinical studies (2).

One reason for the current popularity of unconventional healing methods is the emphasis being placed on consumer participation, the role of the patient in the treatment of his/her own illness. Alternative methods of care focus on the individual with the illness. The term "(W)holistic" is often used synonymously with "alternative," indicating that the focus is not on the disease or the symptom, but on the patient who is host to the illness. This has been aptly stated by great physicians of the past.

Said **Sir William Osler:** "It is more important to know what sort of a patient has the disease than what sort of disease the patient has."

**Claude Bernard** observed: "The germ is nothing—the soil everything."

When asked about his respect for the traditional African Witch Doctor, **Albert Schweitzer** said: "The Witch Doctor succeeds for the same reason all the rest of us succeed. Each patient carries his own doctor inside him. They come to us not knowing that cure. We are at our best when we give the doctor who resides within each patient a chance to work."

Practitioners of various alternative methods often support their techniques with passionate claims. Important to note, however, is that the degree of passion behind such assertions is no measure of the treatment's worth when evaluated in the dispassionate light of scientific investigation. Only thus can we determine how much of mind/body medicine is mind and how much is body.

From the very beginning, magic, medicine, and religion have grown up together. Several thousand years B.C.E. in Asia, the Ayurvedic Medicine of India and Traditional Chinese Medicine were developed without any real knowledge of anatomy or physiology. The early physicians of these countries, like the shamans of many primitive regions, developed their medicine from the philosophy and religious beliefs of the time. Mysterious life forces were believed to flow through hypothesized body channels such as the Chinese *meridians*, conveying *ch'i,* and the *chakras* of India for *prana.* In the 5th Century B.C.E. Hippocratic period, illness was depicted as a disruption in the relationship of the four elements—blood, phlegm and yellow and black bile. Physicians focused their treatments on the individual patient, seeking to bring the four humors into balance. The approach was wholistic and included emphasis on diet, exercise, and meditation, as well as supplication to the gods of healing. It is an enigma that in this day of scientific enlightenment, belief in *chakras, prana, meridians,* and *ch'i* is still accepted unquestioningly by both Eastern and Western physicians.

# Introduction

In the West during the time of Descartes, there was a belief in a mysterious life force. It was believed that the cavities of the brain contained an hypothesized "vital force," a fluid which was pumped through hollow nerves into the muscles, producing their life-like movements. This was known as the "hydraulic theory." This metaphysical theory exploded when, in 1700, Munro showed that nerves were not hollow tubes. This paved the way for Galvani and others to demonstrate the conduction of the nervous impulse by electrical stimulation. Such research tools then became available for a more rational appraisal of the hitherto unexplained mystery of life force.

Through most of the Middle Ages, the mainstay of healing practices remained holistic, including treatments using herbs and amulets. Spiritual and suggestive methods were common practice. It was believed that royalty inherited the power to heal, and at prescribed times, crowds gathered at palaces to be healed by "the King's touch." Cupping, bleeding, and purging added little to the body's own natural healing ability, but this natural healing power persisted, often assisted by placebo magic. Whatever was being done to the patient at the time of natural recovery was, from mere association, given credit for the healing.

There was no knowledge of bacterial infections, and it was widely believed that diseases were caused by unseen spirits. With the development of the microscope, such "spirits" became visible as living "germs." Importantly, in the 17th Century, Thomas Sydenham separated the symptoms of patients into two categories: *1)* pathognomonic – symptoms shared among groups of patients; and *2)* idiosyncratic – symptoms unique to a particular patient. This converted the individual experience of an illness into the group experience of a named disease.

The way was paved for a technologic revolution in medicine. Invention of the stethoscope and the ophthalmoscope in the first half of the 19th Century permitted physicians to objectively hear and see the signs of organ malfunction that the patient was describing as subjective symptoms. In rapid succession came the x-ray, the baumanometer for measuring blood pressure, and a host of laboratory diagnostic technologies. As a result, physicians spent less time talking to patients, and the physical examination became cursory, serving mainly to merely point the physician in the direction of which laboratory or technical diagnostic procedures to order. With expanding medical knowledge, no one person could know in depth all there was to know about each organ or body system, so the patient was divided amongst several medical specialities.

In the late 19th and early 20th Centuries, there were as many homeopathic as allopathic physicians. These two major paradigms of treatment struggled for supremacy. The basic assumptions of homeopathy remained unproven. The American Medical Association espoused scientific medicine and won the day. By the 1930's, the last homeopathic institution, Hahnemann in Philadelphia, had joined the list of allopathic medical schools. Medicine had become truly scientific. As the 20th Century progressed, physicians gained the means for objective representations of illness that bypassed the distortions of the patient's subjective litany of self-observed symptoms. In the 1940's, the diagnostician Tinsley Harrison referred to "the present day tendency toward a five-minute history followed by a five-day barrage of special tests in the hope that the diagnostic rabbit may suddenly emerge from the laboratory hat." In the 70's and 80's, the acme of objectivity had been reached when researchers presented, through the magic of the computer, methods of diagnosis and treatment selection resulting from decision tree algorithms. With this, it became possible for the patient to interact directly with the computer and effectively bypass human interaction with a physician.

While Western scientific medicine was moving in the direction of seeing the patient as a disease rather than as a human being, a swing was also beginning in the opposite direction. Patients began to grumble about doctors not talking to them. Somehow, the derivation of the word "doctor" from the Latin verb *docere*, to teach, was no longer applicable. Physicians seemed to overlook the fact that part of the patient's problem, and perhaps a large factor in the illness, was anxiety about what was going wrong with the body. The media's graphic, televised, and colorful descriptions of cancer, AIDS, and other serious illnesses caused patients' imaginations to work overtime. A little more time to explain the meaning of symptoms and to allay anxiety would have been important. Too often the patient was quickly sent off to the laboratory or dismissed with a hastily written prescription for a drug with frequently unpleasant side effects for which the patient had not been prepared.

Small wonder then that patients began to turn more to those who offered, with great promise, a myriad of alternative therapies, guaranteed to "cure anything from warts to housemaid's knee." As the science fiction writer Ron Hubbard once said, "You find out what the public wants and you give it to them." Some of these alternative therapies, such as chiropractic and osteopathy, had already formed a firm base in the United States. Homeopathy was then resurrected, with schools opening up across the country, this time for non-physicians as well. Herbal medicine manufacturers began rushing to fill orders faster than plant supplies were available. Some ancient practices like astrology, Ayurvedic, and Traditional Chinese Medicine found, as Barnum predicted, that customers were plentiful as long as promises were made. The old attitude prevailed, "Don't bother me with the facts, my mind is already made up!" It became important only that the patient believed in what he/she was being told. If patient and doctor both believe in the efficacy of what is done regardless of the absence of scientific merit, some benefit based upon placebo action can occur. If positive results occur, the technique's reputation will be enhanced and promoted by word of mouth. As long as the human body demonstrates recuperative powers and patients recover and feel better, both conventional and unconventional practices will exist side-by-side.

Another factor in the move toward again looking at the whole person is the ethical one. Beginning in the 1950's, advanced techniques such as the respirator, artificial kidney, and by-pass heart surgery appeared. These could rescue patients from life-threatening physiological failures. Medicine was then faced with a consideration of matters about the quality of life. Right-to-die issues, the choice for abortion and euthanasia, etc., brought forth items of interest to the clergy — the spirit and the soul. Medicine, religion, and law jointly began to debate ethical issues, and hospitals formed medical ethics committees and spoke of the "Patient's Bill of Rights."

All of this has returned the focus of medicine to the whole person. Not only psychiatrists, but even surgeons are beginning to talk about mind/body interaction (3). Group support for cancer patients, including instructions in relaxation, self-hypnosis, and imagery as ways for enhancing anti-tumor killer cell activity are now mentioned in respectable medical journals with referenced articles. The subject of neuro-psychoimmunology — how the mind can strengthen the patient's fight against disease — has gathered 2000 references in medical literature.

"Placebo" was a bad word until the mid-1950's. Now we know that the patient's strong belief can assist in recovery, and in some psychosomatic conditions, can be the curative agent. In the long, dark Middle Ages, placebo medicine was all that accounted for cures by shamans and witches. Now, placebo action is being scientifically investigated, and some believe that it may result from the release of endorphins and other neuropeptides that are part of the essential link between mind and body.

In light of the above, alternative medicine must now be re-examined. Each of its disciplines should in turn be looked at in the same manner that the FDA designates for all new drugs. Only in this way can one see what, if any, factual basis lies beyond the placebo effect. One purpose of this manual is to examine critically the multitude of glorious claims about the efficacy of some of these treatments. It is important to advise the patient of any reasonable probability that a method is based upon biological facts. All physicians should have the knowledge to caution their patients when treatments should be avoided or viewed with suspicion.

Perhaps the word "alternative" will ultimately be replaced by the word "complementary." For since allopathic medicine places increasing emphasis upon primary care, there will be a return to the ways and wisdom of the old family doctor — a physician who again is a teacher, who finds time to talk to the patient, and who integrates the best of those scientifically supported methods of unconventional therapy into everyday modern medical practice.

## REFERENCES

1. Eisenberg, D., et al. (1993). Unconventional medicine in the United States. *New Eng J Med, 328*, 246-252.
2. The politics of alternative medicine. (1994). *Science, 265*, 2000-2002.
3. Seigel, B. (1989). *Peace, love and healing.* New York: Harper & Row.

# ALTERNATIVE MEDICINE
# OR
# MAGICAL HEALING

*"The trick is to know the difference."*

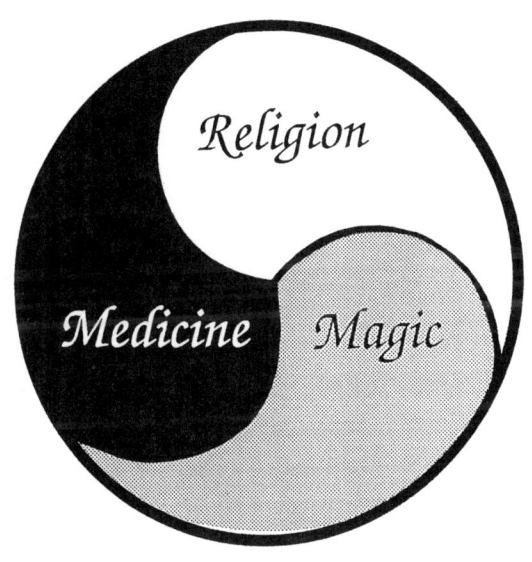

# I

# THE ROOTS OF ALTERNATIVE MEDICINE
## EAST AND WEST

MEDICAL PARADIGMS are models or theories describing systems of belief about healing commonly held by groups of healers. They vary from culture to culture. Worldwide, there are numerous theoretical models that describe different beliefs about how healing works. With today's rapid spread of knowledge, such terms as "Western" and "Eastern" no longer clearly define these different types of practices. Techniques such as traditional Chinese acupuncture and Transcendental Meditation and Yoga from India are now widely practiced in the West, while technical procedures originating in the West such as radiology and electrocardiology are standard practices in many hospitals of the East.

The accepted medical paradigm taught in medical schools of the United States is called "allopathic" or "conventional." Those systems of healing and techniques that are unconventional are commonly termed "alternative." This designation applies not only to techniques and systems of Eastern origin, but also to a large number of other approaches such as chiropractic and homeopathy, which originated in the West.

Although one medical paradigm tends to be commonly held by the majority of healers in any one culture, even within that society individual healers may vary in the model they use to explain what they do to heal their patients. For example, in the case of a successful treatment with acupuncture, one practitioner may believe the treatment is best explained in the metaphysical terms of Traditional Chinese Medicine, while another explains what happens in terms of modern neurophysiology. Despite the vastly different explanations given, the underlying biological alteration and the patient's ability to heal can be the same.

In the beginning, healing practices derived from a combination of magic and religion. Through the centuries and even today, magic, religion, and medicine are woven into everyday healing practices. Shamanism, or magical healing, is still practiced in all parts of the world. It is a polytheistic nature worship, the rituals of which often involve "spirits" and totem animals. As a forerunner of Taoism in the East, it developed from the primitive sorcery of the North Asian people. Typically, the shaman enters into a trance-like state reputedly to become a "messenger," acting as a mediator between the world of ancestral spirits and living humans. Viewed scientifically, the shaman never actually leaves his/her body. "Speaking for departed ancestors" is best interpreted as the reporting of cultural myths and traditions stored in the shaman's memory. Thus, the shaman is able to bring to bear the moral imperatives of past generations upon the problems of today's society as manifested in the illnesses of the patients being treated.

The *wu* of China, the *mansin* of Korea practicing their *kut*, and the *medicine men* of North America healing with sand paintings are all brothers. They use drums, dancing, and animal artifacts to carry out their curative spells. All cultures contain superstitions and other remnants of parapsychological practices that have survived through the ages. Early Oriental shamans practiced arts of divination including the milfoil, which was a casting of sticks of unequal lengths. The patterns they formed became the origin of the 64 hexagrams of the *I Ching,* a most popular Eastern book of prophecy which has been translated and is now available in every bookstore in the West.

African *voodoo* has a belief in spirit possession which has a demonstrated power to heal or even, rarely, to kill. It was brought to America with the slave trade in the 17th-19th Centuries and is still widely practiced in some islands of the Caribbean.

*Qi Gong* is an ancient Chinese shamanist practice of which there are two general types, external *Qi Gong* and internal *Qi Gong*. In external *Qi Gong,* powers claimed to be emitted from the hands of master healers have been likened to infrasonic emissions. The brain wave changes so induced, however, are similar to recent topographical brain maps seen with hypnosis. *Qi Gong* masters in China have recently been labeled as charlatans. An international organization known as the *Committee for the Scientific Investigation of Claims of the Paranormal* (CISCOP) is active in exposing fraudulent healing practices of charlatans who use such methods as astrology, palmistry, and spiritualism to give false medical advice. This group was invited to China in 1988 at the request of China's *Science and Technology Daily* to investigate the growing interest in the paranormal, including external *Qi Gong*. CISCOP conducted experiments in Beijing, Shanghai, and Xian. Under carefully controlled conditions, they examined *Qi Gong* healers and children who claimed clairvoyant powers. The conclusion, documented by video, was that the seeming miracles were accomplished by ordinary means of trickery (1).

In the U.S., *Qi Gong* has caught the fancy of promoters of acupuncture seminars always on the lookout for some new mystery to teach their scientifically naive clientele. Practitioners of external *Qi Gong* have even been joined with practitioners of the equally questionable *O-ring technique* (2). In this, the sensitivity of the *Qi Gong* master detects supposed emanations from a diseased part of the patient's body and produces a weakening of the opposed thumb and finger grip between *Qi Gong* master and the examining physician. Internal *Qi Gong*, on the other hand, is a useful type of mind/body relaxing therapy. Workers at Xian Medical University have produced an amalgamation of East/West medicine in the form of *Qi Gong*-feedback-therapy (QFT), which combines the principle of ancient Chinese internal *Qi Gong* with the techniques of modern Western biofeedback (3).

Religious healings have been and are a universal phenomenon. They are reported in the historical writings of ancient Egypt and Greece, Hindu medicine, the Jewish *Kabbala*, and the medicine of Islam. Christianity, the dominant religion in the West, records in the New Testament of its Bible over 50 miraculous healings performed by Jesus Christ. The philosophical teachings of Descartes in the Middle Ages emphasized "dualism," a separation of the mind from the body. Medicine thereafter increasingly concerned itself solely with treating ailments of the body, leaving the mind and soul to the care of the church. Over the years, various religious healing sects arose and have continued the method of faith healing. It was not, however, until the rise of psychiatry at the beginning of the 20th Century that conventional medicine took a serious look at the functions of the mind and the healing of illness through psychotherapy.

Good evidence exists that a person's strong religious belief can assist healing. Such power should be utilized whenever it is in the patient's best interest. Kua and associates in Singapore (4) have stated that it is important in treatment to take into account the faith, philosophy, and life plan of each patient. Larson (5) has gathered evidence that a strong religious belief can have a positive effect on both mental and physical illness. Such faith healing of the West is like the mind/body medicine of the East. Psychosomatic Medicine, the effect of emotions on illness, had its origin in Western medicine at the turn of the century. From this, increasing interest in psychoimmunology has developed. Mind/body medicine today has thus taken on many faces. Not only is it seen in different forms in Ayurvedic, Buddhist, and traditional Chinese medicines, but in the West it comes under such headings as biofeedback, hypnosis, relaxation response, and imagery.

## Conventional and Unconventional Medicine

Major differences exist between the "conventional" medicine of the West and "alternative" medicine of which major paradigms are derived from traditional Chinese and Ayurvedic practices.

*Conventional medicine* is based upon scientifically supported theories and facts. It tends to be reductionistic, attributing a condition to a single cause. In treatment, the physician takes complete charge, using surgery to remove tumors or powerful pharmaceutical agents to kill invading bacteria, protozoa, or viruses. The treatment is aggressive, swift, and often has side effects. Treatment is usually begun at a late stage in the disease when symptoms are obvious.

*Alternative medicine*, on the other hand, has paradigms based upon the often uncritical acceptance of observations that have been handed down from previous generations of healers. The approach is holistic, assuming multiple causes both within and without the body. The treatment is cooperative in that the patient is strongly urged to participate in his/her own cure and work toward a change in life style. The physician assumes the role of teacher. The treatment is slow, with few side effects. Treatment tends to be given early and is often of a preventive nature, administered before any symptoms occur.

Neither approach is without problems. In the West, many patients believe their doctors are too rushed, don't listen to their complaints, and rely too much on laboratory tests and technical equipment. The effectiveness of drugs and surgery at best is moderate. Treatments are more useful for acute than for chronic conditions. Medical costs are rising. Drugs can have side effects, and the difference between an effective dose and a troublesome dose is small.

Alternative medicine, too, has its problems. Treatments based on metaphysical beliefs rather than experimental facts are subject to myriad interpretations, abuse, and charlatanism. Practitioners are frequently rigidly married to one technique and are therefore known as "hypnotists," "acupuncturists," or "homeopaths." They thus tend to fit all patients to their *Procrustean bed* of one technique of healing and may lack the flexibility to use other treatments when they are more appropriate. As the psychologist Abraham Maslow once said, "If you have only a hammer, all disease is a nail." The subtle effects of preventive treatments are difficult to measure. The herbs of antiquity are often accepted at face value instead of being rigorously tested. All drugs, even herbs, are poison if given in large enough doses.

## Scientizing Traditional Chinese Medicine

Chairman Mao once said, "Ancient Chinese medicine is truly a veritable storehouse." How correct he was. Of the various aspects of Traditional Chinese Medicine, the one that has received the most attention in the West is acupuncture. I first became acquainted with it in Japan before it was introduced to the United States in 1972. I learned and practiced it according to the traditional metaphysical paradigm and, not surprisingly, was able to help many patients. However, as an amateur magician for over 50 years, I am accustomed to searching for the practical secret that lies behind every mystery. The theoretical foundations of traditional Chinese acupuncture certainly presented me with a complex mystery. And so I spent the next few years seeking evidence to support an acceptable Western scientific paradigm for acupuncture (6).

In the three decades following the 60's, much research and great progress was made in understanding the neuro-physiology and neuro-chemistry of the pain nervous system. This opened the door to research, leading to an understanding of the mechanisms underlying acupuncture's effectiveness in controlling pain.

Our own research, published in 1978 (7), demonstrated: (a) that acupuncture was not hypnosis; (b) that electricity was essential to produce a statistically significant relief from experimental pain; and (c) that some acupuncture points had an independent electrical existence. This was in accord with the work of Liu (8) and of Gunn (9) in which it appeared that useful acupuncture points were mainly points where one could gain ready access to the central nervous system, i.e., motor points, points over Golgi tendon organs, and points near major nerves. The construct of an hypothetical meridian system was not necessary to support a scientific understanding of acupuncture. Recently, the work of Han and others (6) has shown that what acupuncture is all about is getting an electrical stimulus into the nervous system for the release of neuropeptides.

**Life Force and Homeostasis**

In the paradigm of ancient Chinese medicine, *meridians* were a kind of three-dimensional route for *ch'i, shue, ting,* and *wei*. The main purpose of acupuncture was to control the circulation of such hypothesized life substances flowing in the *meridians*. Such concepts of life substance as an elusive mysterious body energy have long been the object of concern and dispute among philosophers the world over, and have been described variously. *Elan vitale* was for the French philosopher Henri Bergson (1859-1941) "the creative evolutionary force inherent in all organisms." In most cultures, medicine equates life force with breath. The old Jewish/Christian scriptures state that after creating man, "God breathed into his nostrils" and, as stated in the Book of Job, it was "the breath of the Almighty" that gave man both life and understanding. Some believe that the soul enters the body with the first breath. Certainly, death begins with the last. In ancient Greek medicine it was known as *pneuma*. In China it is *ch'i*. In the Ayurvedic medicine of India, it is *prana* and is therapeutically manipulated by yogic exercises designed to drive the life force upward through the seven mystical *chakras*.

When I was in medical school 50 years ago, we looked for answers to life's driving forces in either the biochemistry or neurophysiology of the central nervous system. This was a research battle between the "soups" and the "sparks." The debate was which paradigm was more important, the chemical or the electrical aspect in bodily processes. As a researcher in the field of electroencephalography, I felt the "sparks" were most important and acknowledged a deep debt to the English school of neurophysiology. Advances in neurobiology anticipated recent publications by Nordenstrom (10) and Becker (11), who have pointed out the importance of minute electromagnetic processes in body functions. At that time, I was intrigued by Burr's description of energy forces surrounding all living things (12) and by Leao's research on spreading depression, a slow change in polarity measurable on the surface of the brain (13). Our group looked for these slowly moving potentials and we reported a study of D.C. brain waves with frequencies measured in minutes and hours occurring after a brief strong electrical stimulus across the human scalp (14). Perhaps these long-lasting D.C. potential changes may account for some of the observations proposed to support the ancient theory of life force.

Recently, the focus of neurophysiologic research has been on the synapse, neurotransmitters, and membrane phenomena. The new biology has given us a completely different concept of the cell membrane, an understanding of the importance of calcium channels, second messenger systems, DNA, and genome mapping. Worldwide, researchers are still focused upon the "decade of the brain," and who knows what wonders the "soup" and "spark" scientists will reveal next.

Modern biologists frequently define life force by listing the five characteristics necessary to a living organism. These are: *1) order* (the precise arrangement of structural units); *2) adaptations* (structures and activities that allow the organism to better adapt to its environment); *3) metabolism* (the chemical breakdown, conversion and use of energy-rich compounds); *4) movement* (the self-generated motion of an individual or its parts); and *5) responsiveness* (the tendency of an organism to sense and react to its surroundings (15).

There is a saying that "the whole is greater than the sum of its parts." Thus, within one's body, energy and bodily functions derive from the interaction of the several individual organ systems. Without an understanding of the physiology and biochemistry of each of these parts of the system, however, the function and dysfunction of the total body remain a metaphysical mystery.

Western medical scientists have laid a physiological foundation for understanding mind/body medicine. Some of those who made important contributions were:

(a) Claude Bernard, who described homeostasis (16);

(b) Walter Cannon, whose book *Wisdom of the Body* describes how the total body functions to preserve the human being (17);

(c) Hans Selye, who described in detail how the various body systems come into play when the body is subjected to stress (18);

(d) Stanley Cobb, who wrote about built-in body survival mechanisms (19); and

(e) Walter Hess, whose classic work described the functions of the hypothalamus and thalamus as centers of communication for the various body parts (20).

These scientists and others have laid the foundation for an understanding of the physiology and biochemistry of homeostasis, the mechanism by which the body maintains a steady state between extremes. These are Western contributions to the biological basis of what in the East is seen as mysterious mind/body medicine.

On the clinical side: early in this century in the West, the doctrine of psychosomatic medicine gave promise of integrating mind/body concerns as a part of allopathic medicine. Its emphasis was directed primarily toward a search for the psychological factors that caused or influenced certain somatic illnesses. The "holy seven" illnesses of psychosomatic medicine which are most often cited as having an emotional causation or aggravation are: bronchial asthma, rheumatoid arthritis, ulcerative colitis, essential hypertension, neurodermatitis, thyrotoxicosis, and duodenal ulcer. Practitioners of psychosomatic medicine emphasize that psychosocial factors such as environmental and family stresses, poor coping behaviors, and job tension are often major factors in such illnesses. Science is no respecter of hallowed theories. With the discovery of *Helicobacter pylori* as the bacterial agent responsible for peptic ulcer the importance of stress causation comes into question. Hence, the valance of mind/body medicine is not a fixed entity.

The paradigm of mind/body medicine in the Eastern sense of the word has assumed increasing importance with the growing interest in alternative medicine. Thus, Western physicians-in-training are urged to spend more time searching for significant causative psychosocial factors and fitting the treatment to individual needs and personality. Research efforts in the area of psychoneuroimmunology elucidate how the body's immune system reacts to both external and internal stressors.

## Herbology

Increasingly obvious is that the body is neither biochemical or physiological, but that the two are closely interwoven. Such holism has long been recognized in Eastern medicine. Traditional Chinese Medicine's classic work, the *Nei Ching,* differentiates *Ling Shu* — treatment by acupuncture — from the *Su Wen*, which ranges over the general field of medicine and includes exercise and the use of herbal substances. The Chinese *Pen Tsao* ("Great Herbs"), written about 3000 B.C.E., mentions the use of 365 drugs, including *Papaver Sominiferum,* the opium poppy, and *Ma Huang* for bronchial problems. This crude horsetail-like plant grew profusely along the Great Wall and was examined by the Emperor Shen Nung 5,000 years ago. Its active principle *ephedra* has become the basic medicine for bronchial problems all over the world.

In China, as in other countries where folk medicine is prevalent, the use of herbs is not limited to traditional medical practitioners. Self-medication is widely practiced. Secret prescriptions from the ancestors *(Cho-toan pi-hng)* are handed down from generation to generation. Neighbors prescribe for neighbors, and independent pharmacies and herb stores act as the first line of treatment by both diagnosing illness and prescribing remedies. Promoted by the large international drug companies, Western medicines are increasingly appearing on Eastern drugstore shelves, among the over 1,800 herbs listed in the Chinese pharmacopoeia. Today, many of these are the subject of careful scientific study.

One of the earliest records of the use of herbs was from clay tablets left by the Sumerians dating from 4,000 B.C.E. Another, the *Ebers Papyrus*, found between the knees of an Egyptian mummy, is a 68-foot scroll containing references to over 800 plant and animal remedies. In India, the 4,500 year old *Rig Veda* listed 67 medicinal plants. Islamic medicine, as practiced by Rhazes and Avicenna, followed the doctrines of Hippocrates and Galen and, like Ayurvedic medicine, classified drugs according to such qualities as "hot" and "cold," and matched them to the personality characteristics of each patient.

In Europe, folk remedies of native herbs were a mainstay of treatment throughout the Dark Ages (5th-11th Centuries). Formulae for the use of drugs became mixed with the ideas of superstition and magic practiced by witches. These early practitioners of alternative medicine were mostly women who were brutally persecuted during the Inquisition by the male-dominated church. Belief in astrology was prominent, and prescriptions containing metals were associated with astrological signs. William Withering, an English physician, applied the first scientific approach to herbal treatment in 1785. He carefully described the symptoms of his patients, giving the indications and doses of foxglove, the active principle of which is digitalis. This is still a major cardiac medicine. Thus, one can see that herbal remedies, both crude and refined, have had a long history of use worldwide, both East and West. They are useful and potent treatments for many illnesses.

It is unfortunate that the term "homeopathy" is often used interchangeably with "herbology." Homeopathy is based on several questionable hypotheses. These include the "law of the infinitesimal," a belief that the weaker the dilution, the stronger the medicine — even to the point at which, in accord with Avagadro's law, the solution contains no single molecule of the drug. Homeopaths have resurrected the ancient belief of *similia similibus curentur*, that "like cures like." For example, herbs are prescribed because they resemble the organ to be treated, or because when given to a volunteer, they have been found to produce the symptoms of the disease to be treated. For example, drugs that cause fever are used by homeopaths to treat the symptom of fever, whereas general medical experience shows that not all fevers are beneficial, and some can even kill (21).

The broader term "herbology" indicates a less doctrinaire practice which, devoid of metaphysical beliefs, can best serve patients worldwide. It encompasses the scientific study of natural herbs and can be combined with the development and use of newer synthetic drugs as seen in the West. Herbology is increasingly practiced around the world and by naturopaths and chiropractors in the United States. As *Kampo* medicine, it is practiced by an estimated 70% of Japanese physicians. It is central to medical practice in Africa and is a mainstay of the Mexican *curanderos*. In Europe, "phytotherapy" is a term used for the widely accepted practice of herbal medicine.

A report of a recent conference held in London (22) pointed to increasing interest in the West in Chinese and Ayurvedic herbology. One problem discussed was the great variance in the amount of training among those practicing herbal medicine. The participants at the conference ranged from pharmacologists and physicians of the Western allopathic tradition to those who followed European, Chinese, and Indian herbal paradigms. The report indicated that a consensus was reached about several matters of common concern. Participants agreed that better standards and regulations were needed to ensure safety and uniformity of labeled herbal preparations, and that training should be offered to guarantee higher standards and to limit practice to persons thoroughly trained in the use of herbs.

Natural plants are a major resource for modern pharmaceutical manufacturers. Almost 25% of drugs used in Western medicine were first identified as plants. Many of these have been around for a long time and, like digitalis, are still the drugs of choice in their chosen areas. Over half of the top 250 pharmaceutical companies have shown increasing interest in medicinal plants and have research programs in this area. India and China have active programs seeking to identify the essential components of their natural drug remedies.

Yet today, less than 10% of the estimated 250,000 flowering plant species of the world have been examined scientifically for their medical potential. A danger is that with the accelerating destruction of the rain forests of the world, some 60,000 of these plants will become extinct in the next 50 years. This fact should focus the attention of all of us upon the worldwide problems of pollution, the population explosion, and destruction of the world's natural resources.

**Impediments to Evaluation of Treatment Efficacy**

In 1978, WHO officially recognized that traditional medicine could well play a role in achieving the goal of "health for all by the year 2000." Western medicine, despite its demonstrated effectiveness in treating and preventing many illnesses that have long plagued developing nations, is not an appropriate and available substitute acceptable for the 80% of the world's population who depend upon traditional practices concordant with their culture. Often the scientific differences in methodology are not as important as the differences in spiritual and moral beliefs. Traditional healing methods are based on and are highly dependent upon local social/cultural, philosophical, and religious customs. Such practices have stood the test of time, meeting over the centuries the medical needs of the world's burgeoning populations. Thus, WHO has encouraged the support and growth of the traditional practices that appear to have a proven intrinsic worth.

In the West today, there is increasing emphasis on the evaluation of quality of care, outcome data, and cost effectiveness. Although ultimately essential for judging treatment effectiveness, these measures would be difficult to apply to indigenous folk medicine. The theoretical explanations for many alternative practices of both Eastern and Western origin are colored by magical thinking. This tendency to base behavior on what we believe rather than on demonstrated facts is a great hindrance to any evaluation of the real effectiveness of such treatments. Semantic errors include:

- •PALEOLOGIC THINKING, implying causality simply by reason of association in time or place;

- •RETROSPECTIVE FALSIFICATION, the recalling of events as we wish they had happened rather than how they actually happened;

- •AUTO-SUGGESTION, convincing ourselves of what we wished to believe in the first place, regardless of the facts;

- •DOGMATISM, a closed mind not influenced by what actually occurs.

Scientific thinking is based on facts obtained from study, research, and carefully recorded observations. In the field of medicine, the answers are not always clear. For example, it is estimated that up to 80% of illnesses are self-limited. Also, the placebo factor must be taken into account in every treatment evaluation.

The best research is done with both observers and patients blinded and assigned randomly, and with control groups matched to patients and receiving look-alike placebo treatments. There is much that could be gained by such an approach to the study of alternative treatment methods.

Of increasing importance in evaluating the effectiveness of both Western and Eastern healing techniques is a consideration of the **placebo** effect. Placebo response, the positive effect of the doctor's opinion upon the patient, accounts for 30-60% of the healing power of any treatment. Research findings, including work with nalaxone, suggest that the placebo reaction may possibly be related to immune function and mediated through neuropeptides.

Placebo effects are of particular importance in evaluating procedures of alternative medicine whose proclaimed benefits have seldom been checked against standard double-blind research procedures.

Although science has made marvelous contributions to our understanding of the world, this does not mean that all Western treatment techniques are preferable. One should not expect all of the results from Western research laboratories to reveal final truths. Science, being a product of human effort, has its faults, errors, and imperfections. Research findings are often only "straw men," useful hypotheses until further research disproves and replaces them. Many beliefs that I acquired in medical school a scant 50 years ago have been abandoned or have been greatly changed by newer medical knowledge. Thus, as new technologies develop, the old paradigms change.

The fact that scientific medicine is the only form of medicine practiced in many parts of the West does not mean that it is the best form of medicine. Complicated technical procedures are preferable only when simpler alternative methods fail to demonstrate equally good results or the same results without side effects.

**Medical Paradigms—Alternative or Complimentary?**

*So what can alternative practices contribute to our conventional system of Western medicine?* Recommendation for use in clinical practice methods to strengthen the body's own defense mechanisms. Through mind/body healing methods, one can strengthen the energetic forces important for the communication and integration of the body's many separate organ systems. This knowledge should be applied clinically to emphasize a more holistic and preventive type of medicine. Treatments should be formulated while taking into consideration individual differences between patients, despite categorical diagnoses. As is common in Chinese and Ayurvedic medicine, the individual treatment plan formulated for each patient should include proper diet, exercise, a healthy life style, meditation, therapeutic physical practices, and (where appropriate) the employment of natural herbs.

*What can scientific Western medicine offer to the traditional practices that make up the bulk of medical care in developing nations?* Research methodology and the clinical application of the results of scientific discoveries. There are new life-saving diagnostic technologies such as the CAT scan and NMRI, and newer pharmacological agents for fighting infections.

Medical advances arising from biotechnology, while not yet available, are exciting. Based on findings of the Human Genome Project, medical care in the future will be customized to each individual by testing the patient's DNA against a micro-chip with picographs of diagnostic DNA—an advanced scientific model of the individualization of patient treatment that has been a tradition in the practice of Eastern mind/body medicine.

Scientists are involved in cutting-edge work in genetics, leading to biological preparations specific for enhancing immune functions in the battle against AIDS and neoplasms. In third world countries, recent genome initiatives are tackling the big killers, including *Dracunculiasis, Malaria, Schistosomiasis*, and others. Such diseases in Africa, India, and much of Asia account for well over half of the total burden of morbidity and mortality of those populations. Advances in computer and telecommunications have now linked isolated rural practitioners to high tech medical centers. Such technologies could readily make the diagnostic tests of scientific medicine available to folk healers in third world countries.

## Conclusion

How does one integrate the two paradigms of medicine, East and West? The answer is not to substitute Western medicine in the East. This is neither philosophically nor economically practical any more than substituting Eastern medicine in the West where it is socio/culturally incongruent. However, the goal of integration can and will be accomplished.

The answer is to be found in research efforts such as those demonstrated by the WHO-sponsored East-West Medical Research Institute of Kung Hee University in Soeul, Korea. Recognition of the importance of research on Alternative Medicine has also been shown in the United States by the establishment of an Office of Alternative Medicine in the National Institutes of Health. In April 1994, the European Parliament adopted a proposal calling for the provision of complementary medicine within social security systems, incorporation of complementary medicines in the European pharmacopoeia, and a research budget of 10 million *ecus* (about 7.5 million pounds) a year for five years (23).

A major impediment to the worldwide acceptance of these valuable treatment methods is the aura of mystery that surrounds an approach foreign to Western scientific thinking. Most physicians trained in the West are unwilling to spend the many hours necessary to master the basic metaphysical and cosmological concepts of Traditional Chinese and Ayurvedic medicine. This hindrance can be overcome by what I like to term the "scientization" of traditional techniques.

A few examples exist. Herbert Benson of Harvard Medical School studied the yogic methods of Ayurvedic medicine. From this, he developed the *Relaxation Response* technique (24). This Americanized version of the ancient Indian practice of Transcendental Meditation is accepted widely and used in the West. Research workers at Xian Medical University have combined Internal *Qi Gong* with Biofeedback to create the East/West technique of QFT, *Qi Gong Feedback Treatment* (3). Many studies worldwide seek to bring order and regulation into the vast storehouse of herbal medicine. Examples are ongoing research efforts on apparently useful remedies such as *Ginko biloba*.

My own experience with scientized acupuncture has been salutary. Teaching this technique from the standpoint of neurophysiology obviates the necessity for hundreds of hours of study to gain a background in the theories of Traditional Chinese Medicine. Formerly, students were turned off by the metaphysical and cosmological interpretations of this treatment method. Now they readily accept a simplified acupuncture technique that can be taught in a single afternoon session.

It is increasingly important for traditional doctors to be familiar with modern diagnostic techniques and understand about the treatment methods used by Western physicians. It is just as important for Western physicians to understand what traditional healers do. Not that they should spend long hours mastering the metaphysical philosophies currently considered essential for the practices of Traditional Chinese and Ayurvedic medicine. They must, however, know about these things if research technologies are to have an impact. Especially important is recognition of the socio-cultural beliefs basic to the patients we treat.

In the United States, the family doctor is looked upon as furnishing the most cost-effective level of medical care. Medical schools are now increasing the number of family practice doctors in training. These are the physicians who should learn the techniques of both Eastern and Western medicine.

Thus, there are indications that these two medical paradigms, conventional and unconventional, can be melded into a single system of medicine that is neither frozen in technology nor lost in metaphysics, a medicine that is comprehensive, in which treatment techniques are not alternative, but rather complementary to one another, thus offering the best of care for the ills of all humankind.

## REFERENCES

1. Kurtz, P., et al. (1988). Testing psi claims in China: Visit by a CSICOP delegation. *Skeptical Inquirer, 12*, 364-375.
2. Omura, Y. (1989). Meridians and internal organs, etc. *Acup and Electro-Ther Res J, 14*, 155-186.
3. Li, Y., et al. (1989). A comparative study on experiences of qigong and biofeedback therapy. (Proceedings of the Second International Conference on Qigong). Xian, China: Tian Ze Press.
4. Kua, E.H.; Che, P.H.; & Ko, S.M. (1993). Spirit possession and healing among Chinese psychiatric patients. *Acta Psychiatr Scand, 88*, 447-450.
5. Larson, D., & Larson, S. (1991). Religious commitment and health: Valuing the relationship. *Second Opinion, Faith and Ethics, 17*, 26-40.
6. Ulett, G.A. (1992). *Beyond Yin and Yang: How acupuncture really works.* (1992). St. Louis: Warren H. Green.
7. Parwatikar, S., et al. (1978). Acupuncture, hypnosis and experimental pain: I study with volunteers. *Acup and Electro-Ther Res J, 3*, 161-190.
8. Liu, Y.H.; Varela, M.; & Oswald, R. (1975). Correspondence between some motor points and acupuncture loci. *Amer J Chin Med, 3*, 347-358.
9. Gunn, C.C. (1978). Motor points and motor lines. *Am J Acup, 6*, 55-58.

10. Nordenstrom, B. (1991). Bioelectrical circuits in the body. *Frontier Perspectives, 2*, 16-18.
11. Becker, R. (1990). *Cross currents: The promise of electro-medicine; the perils of electropollution.* Los Angeles: Jeremy P.Tarcher.
12. Burr, H.S. (1932). Electro-dynamic theory of development suggested by studies of proliferation rates in brain of amblystoma. *J Comp Neurol, 56*, 347-371.
13. Leao, A. (1941).Steady potential fields and neurone activity. *J Neuro-physiol, 4*, 438-455.
14. Goldring, S., et al. (1950). Initial survey of slow potential changes obtained under resting conditions and incident to convulsive therapy. *EEG Clin Neurophysiol, 2*, 297-308.
15. Hopson, J. (1989). *The nature of life.* New York: W.W. Norton.
16. Bernard, C. (1880). *Lecons de physiologie experimentel appliquee a la medicine au College de France.* Paris, France: J. E. Bailliere et fils.
17. Cannon, W. (1932). *Wisdom of the body.* New York: W.W. Norton.
18. Selye, H. (1956). *The stress of life.* New York: McGraw Hill.
19. Cobb, S. (1941). *Foundations of neuropsychiatry.* Baltimore: Williams & Wilkins.
20. Hess, W. (1969). *Hypothalamus and thalamus, experimental documentation.* Stuttgart: Thieme.
21. Mackowiak, P. (1994). Fever: blessing or curse? A unifying hypothesis. *Ann Int Med, 120*, 1037-1040.
22. Atherton, D. (1994). Towards the safer use of traditional remedies. *Brit Med J, 308*, 673-674.
23. Fisher, P., & Ward, A. (1994). Complimentary medicine in Europe. *Brit Med J, 309*, 107-111.
24. Benson, H. T. (1975). *The relaxation response.* New York: Avon Books.

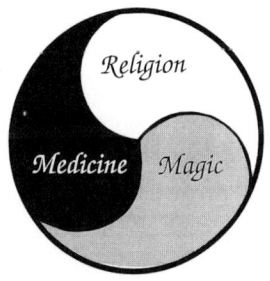

# II

# HUMAN PROPENSITY FOR MAGIC AND MYSTERY

FROM THE VERY BEGINNING, magic, religion, and healing have been so closely bound together that they are often indistinguishable from one another. Through the centuries their paths frequently diverged, but just as frequently again intertwined. Janet, a famous French psychologist, once said of Grandmother's hat that although it fell out of fashion, it should not be discarded for it will again return to fashion's favor. Recurring magical themes are typical of both religion and healing as they are resurrected by promoters of New Age hype.

Humans are blessed with a great curiosity. The search for answers from childhood on is a constant asking of "why?" The desire for explanations is never outgrown. This is exemplified by the ceaseless efforts of inventors and scientific researchers who pose questions and then seek answers to their own hypotheses about natural and observed phenomena. Their studies have resulted in a massive accumulation of facts that has outstripped library shelves and entered the world of computers via the "information highway." This explosion of scientific knowledge has resulted in the advanced technology and comforts of today's world. Despite the fact that holistic healing techniques have been around for centuries, it is the recent advances in medicine and public health that have brought about a doubling of life expectancy since the beginning of this century.

We are living in a time of abundant knowledge, which is available to explain most of the natural phenomena that for generations mystified humankind. What for centuries was attributed to the capricious action of gods and spirits is now very simply explained in high school physics and biology textbooks. Lightening is no longer Jove's thunderbolt hurled to earth. It is now understood as an electromagnetic phenomenon. Still today, thousands, perhaps the majority of persons in even the most advanced civilized nations, worship at the altar of faith rather than of fact. There is a continuance of the childhood belief in magic and in the existence of tooth fairies, ghosts, and Santa Claus. Since the end of World War II, there has been continued growth in the credence and hope for mystical cures at the hands of charismatic religious healers and the eager purveyors of the fanciful healing rituals of alternative medicine.

Faith or belief can be a conviction or certainty in something for which there is a lack of sufficient evidence to define a numerical or rational probability. Examples abound in superstitious rituals to ward off evil or to promote good fortune. Like the behavior of compulsive neurotics who perform their rituals to control anxiety, Taoist monks spin their prayer wheels endlessly to invoke the good will of the Gods. So, too, gamblers in Las Vegas fondle their lucky pieces in a vain attempt to control the fall of the dice.

**Magic**

A pervasive belief in magic is ever-present in the human mind. In the 60's, a prominent tobacco company mounted an advertising campaign which exposed some stage illusions presented by popular vaudeville magicians. The catch phrase was "It's fun to be fooled, it's more fun to know." For many, the exact opposite is true, as "the mysterious" retains its attraction only when answers are unknown. The tendency to believe and use mysterious explanations for common events is found in all cultures. Historically, the belief systems of both healing and religion reveal an unbroken path from the magic of ancient shamanism to the healings of some modern day television evangelists and charismatic New Age healers.

As emphasized by Carl Sagan (1), pseudoscience is a worldwide phenomenon. In the U.S., the CIA wasted 20 million dollars of taxpayer's money on its Stargate program. This was a futile 20-year race with the Soviets, hoping to find ways to utilize parapsychology as a cold war weapon. Astrology is common among the "godmen" of India. *Qi Gong* witchcraft is practiced in China. Witches are still burned in Africa.

Algeria has 10,000 soothsayers, half with government licenses. The "psychic surgery" hoax continues in the Philippines, and in Thailand, diseases are treated with pills manufactured from pulverized sacred scriptures.

While magic has long been a part of shamanism and witchcraft, it has also been a form of entertainment. Illustrations of early Roman feasts and celebrations show jugglers performing simple magic tricks.

Romano (2) has reviewed the early portrayal of magicians by artists in the Middle Ages and before. Paintings by German artist Joseph von Ulm (1404 A.D.), Hieronymus Bosch (1453-1516), Pieter Bruegel the Elder (1525-1569), and French cartoonists Daumier (1808-1879) and Cham (1818-1879) portrayed the magician as a symbol of not only entertaining deception but also hokum and fraud. These artists illustrated their work with demons such as those described by witches as being under their control by means of their herbal and magical potions. The magical trick, the "cups and balls" became a symbol used to illustrate how the government manipulated society.

Some of these magicians or "jugglers" kept the attention of the audience while an accomplice picked their pockets. Magicians were thus both entertainers and charlatans whose clients were pawns to be relieved of their money by trickery. They were forerunners of the riverboat gamblers who in turn foreshadowed the current craze for riverboat casinos.

Magic tricks have been used not only to amuse but also to influence, especially primitive people. The story of Robert Houdin's experience in Algiers in 1855 is of interest (3). The French were having trouble controlling the unruly desert tribes who were unduly influenced by the native conjurors or *Marabouts*. Robert Houdin, the most famous European conjuror of the time, was sent by the French government to Algiers, where he put on an impressive magical performance including the famous trick of catching a bullet in his mouth from a gun fired at an apple held before his face. This so mystified the Arab chieftains that they capitulated to the French government's demands. It is said that Eric Weiss took the name of Robert Houdin, adding an "i" in order to make the name "Houdini." He thought this indicated that he was a modern version of the famous Robert Houdin.

During the heyday of vaudeville and chataquas, the famous Houdini was followed by many other stage magicians and illusionists whose names became household words. These include Thurston, the Blackstones senior and junior, Douglas Henning, David Copperfield, Sigfried and Roy, and many others. Despite the marvels of radio, television, computers, and household gadgets operated by electricity, magnetism, and electronics, interest in sleight-of-hand performances, stage illusions, and conjuring have continued to grow. Throughout the world today, thousands of performers, amateur and professional, belong to such fraternal associations as the International Brotherhood of Magicians. They display their legerdemanic skills at night clubs, churches, school auditoriums, conventions, and elsewhere.

Magic and mystery—through the ages and still today—have a great appeal to all humans. This love of magic has enabled legitimate conjurors to amass great fortunes through their shows of illusion which appeal to audiences throughout the world.

On the seamier side, the widespread belief in magic and mystery has proven equally fascinating and financially rewarding for those who exploit the universal belief in faith healing. The Elmer Gantrys and numerous T.V. evangelists such as the Bakers and Jerry Falwell appeal to viewers worldwide and collect tax-free millions to support their "radio churches" and their own luxurious life-styles. It should be mentioned here that the true founders of legitimate religions—Christ, Mohammed, Luther, Buddha, and others—have always lived for the benefit of humankind only, and were themselves satisfied to live austere lives.

The "magicians of alternative medicine" use as bait to attract their patients such mysterious lures as an ability to command healing by strange body energies. That these have no demonstrated basis in fact only enhances their deceptive attraction. While it might appear that the less educated and superstitious would be prime targets for such treatments, studies in the U.S. and Canada have shown that affluent and well-educated persons patronize these holistic healers (4). One explanation is that Medicare, most HMO's, and health insurance companies do not pay for unorthodox treatments. Thus, the wealthy can best afford such questionable ministrations that last year added another $10 billion to what the U.S. spent for health care.

As there are no *meridians* or anatomically demonstrated *chakras*, and as body energy is a nebulous concept probably unrelated to useful healing, what is it that these medical magicians are selling? Despite mystical theories, the healing accomplishments of alternative practitioners can be explained by their use of practices more commonly known as good preventive medicine. All these practitioners stress good diet, vitamins, exercise, and forms of relaxation. The other stuff is simply attractive window dressing, the gimmick or bait that attracts the victim. For cost effectiveness, the hygienic methods of preventive medicine could be taught in grade school without the magical trappings.

But as long as there are persons with chronic diseases that do not respond well to the usual methods of allopathic medicine, there will always be ready customers for health-care charlatans. It is not, however, that charlatans are always outright frauds. Many honestly believe that what they do is legitimate healing, for they, like their patients, are susceptible to the wiles and fascination of magic.

Yes, it is fun to be fooled by magic. However, when that magic concerns health, it is far better to know the facts!

**Shamanism**

The shaman, or medical man, was a central figure in religious/medical healing ceremonies dating back some 20,000 years in Europe and northern Asia, spreading to the Eskimos and to North and South America (5). Shamanic healers are still found the world over. They continue as a social heritage among the American Indians and others, even for persons living in societies where modern medical methods are known and practiced. The World Health Organization encourages such traditional healers to continue their work while training them in more modern practices of hygiene and midwifery.

The word "shaman" derives from the Tunguso-Manchurian word *saman,* which means "one who knows." Often marked by some physical abnormality such as an extra finger or toe or epileptic seizures, the shaman is selected at youth and apprenticed to the profession over a period of many years. It is believed that the shaman has inherited the soul of a previous shaman or that of a strong totem animal.

The shaman typically heals as an intermediary (psychopomp) with the spirit world. Invoking a trance, he/she travels to the spirit world and returns with healing power.

Typically, the trance is produced by singing, chanting, dancing, and drumming. Drums are made from the hides of important totem animals. The shaman collects various healing artifacts — parts of animals, birds, colorful stones, and the like — that are also used to decorate the costumes and headdresses worn during the ceremonies.

The shaman is responsible as keeper of the tribe's cultural heritage and healing knowledge told through chants and ceremonies. Healing ceremonies are long and involve not only the patient and immediate family but often the whole community. The ways of shamanic healing are imbedded in community belief systems to which patients are exposed from childhood. They have a strong belief in the magic of the shaman, and hence there is a strong placebo effect. Participation in an intense community ceremony boosts the patient's self confidence and reaffirms belief. It is proposed that rhythmic drumming, the heartbeat that brings the tribe together, can stimulate the flow of healing neuropeptides and thus strengthen the immune response.

The art of healing is a way of life to the native American Indians. All Indian healing is closely connected to Mother Earth and is inseparable from day-to-day existence. The whole environment — earth, trees, animals, sun, and sky — is involved in the healing process. All of nature is sacred; every animal, rock, and plant is believed to contain a spirit. The relationship of humankind to the environment and to healing is one of respect and appreciation of the power held within. All forces of creation are thus woven dynamically into a harmonious whole.

A special relationship exists between the medicine man or woman and the tools utilized in the healing process. The feather of an eagle is important because the eagle can fly high and is a messenger of truth between humans and the Great Spirit in the sky. Crystals are important because they transmit energy, and colors take on a special significance.

The Indian's "bible" consists of elaborate ceremonies held in the tribe's memory and is recalled in the form of songs, chants, and dances. Thus, from early childhood, the knowledge and firm belief in the healing powers of the medicine man and his ceremonies are a part of the individual and community belief systems.

Navajo Indian society well demonstrates a type of holistic medicine. It is a healing system interwoven with the entire culture and environment, becoming an essential part of the mind, body, and spirit.

Once he is selected in childhood and destined to become the tribe's medical man, the prospective healer is rigorously and painfully trained. Until 1960, there was no written Navajo language, so all details of the elaborate healing ceremonies of that tribe had to be committed to memory. Thus, after years of apprenticeship, the medicine man often did not begin healing practices until the fourth decade of life.

Typically, the center of healing in the Indian village is the hogan, a round or 6- or 8-sided structure, importantly without corners. A simple opening faces east. This building, known as the "sweat lodge," is found in each village, and by raising body temperature, plays an important role in healing and purification ceremonies. These ceremonies last typically from one to nine days, depending upon the nature and seriousness of the illness. Mental illnesses may require nine days.

The initial ceremonies are for purification and begin with a dance, at which time masks are worn. The healing part of the ceremony then proceeds with the making of a sand painting on the dirt floor of the hogan. The painting is made from different colored sands and pulverized rocks and is created by assistants under the direction of the medicine man. There are only a few basic forms of sand painting, with minor variations. The designs are elaborate, with figures and symbols signifying magic and beliefs from the dim past.

The medicine man passes his power into the painting. The patient then sits on a designated part of the painting in order to absorb the healing power therefrom. After the patient has been sitting on the painting for about 30 minutes, the medicine man pronounces his blessing. The sand painting, having done its healing work, is swept up into a blanket and is scattered to the winds. The healing is over.

In some parts of the country where plant growth is abundant, native Indian tribal medicines are made from the various herbs of the region. Cactus grows in the desert, and peyote, obtained from the dried upper part of the mescal cactus, produces an intoxicated state that is sometimes a part of the ceremony. The smoking of tobacco is also a common practice in all Indian ceremonies.

Viewed psychologically, the ceremony involves: identification, transference, confession, extinction of anxiety, and suggestions that are supportive of already existing beliefs. The healing is thus an example of bringing the body into homeostatic balance. In Navajo, the term *hochogi* comes closest to expressing the concept of disease. It is translated as "unpleasant condition" or possibly "stress." Curing, then, is a return to *hozhogi*, meaning "pleasant condition" or "wellness." Among the Navajo, if the medicine man is strong and lives an exemplary life, he is said to "walk his talk" and is often the most powerful person in the tribe.

Because shamanic healing involves the whole community and particularly members of the extended family, there is much environmental support and a reconstitution of ego defenses. Such healing ceremonies have a strong impact on mind/body interactions and may strengthen the immune reaction through mechanisms of psycho-neuro-immunology. In current parlance, the psychiatrist heals using a **bio-psycho-social** approach. In shamanic healing, a fourth factor is added, making the method truly an example of **bio-psycho-social-spiritual** healing.

An example of a contemporary shaman is Edgar Cayce (6). He was born in Hopkinsville, Kentucky in 1880. At the age of six, he reported to his parents that he could see "visions." By sleeping with his head on his books, his "photographic memory" allowed him to absorb the contents of the books. This gift faded and he graduated from only the 7th grade. When he was 21 and working as a salesman for a wholesale stationary company, he developed a paralysis of his throat muscles. Physicians failed to cure him and he had a friend help him enter the type of hypnotic trance that he had used with his schoolbooks when he was a child. In this self-induced trance, he perceived the proper therapy of medication and manipulation that "cured" his condition.

After this, he began to give readings for persons with various illnesses. He would give his readings while lying relaxed on a couch seemingly asleep, but talking. During these trance states, he supposedly received medical information from "messengers in the spirit world." If a patient was in the room during his trance, he might talk to him or her as though he/she were in a former reincarnation. A secretary or his wife sat nearby, recording his utterances until he awakened from his trance.

A group of local physicians utilized Edgar Cayce's unique talents to diagnose their own patients. It was soon discovered that he only needed the name and address of a distant patient and he could, by seemingly telepathic means, discover the nature of the affliction and would recommend a treatment. Such simple home remedies as castor-oil packs were commonly recommended. It was enigmatic that this relatively unschooled man with no medical training and apparently no contact with medical texts could make difficult medical diagnoses and treatments.

Until his death at the age of 65 in 1945, he had given over 14,000 readings. His home in Virginia Beach is now the Edgar Cayce Foundation, the Association for Research and Enlightenment, (ARE). His readings constitute one of the largest collections of psychic perception ever to emanate from a single individual. Along with relevant correspondence and reports, they have been cross-indexed under thousands of subject headings and placed at the disposal of writers, psychologists, and researchers of holistic healing.

While shamanic healing depends on cultural factors that induce individual beliefs, the mystical behavior of the shaman is the strong instigating factor. How the shaman performs his/her "magic act" is of interest and has been the subject of several various hypotheses. In all shamanic healings, both ancient and modern, the shaman creates an altered state of consciousness during which he/she exhibits hallucinatory-type behavior. Wright (7) has reviewed the literature that posits possible neurophysiological correlations for such behaviors. Endorphins, hallucinogens, and genetic factors could all play a role. Studies of shamanic-type meditation are known to produce EEG patterns with increased abundance, voltage, and a synchrony of alpha and theta activity. Rhythmic auditory stimuli such as shamanic singing, chanting, and drumming may produce auditory driving of the EEG. Temporal lobe transients and disinhibition might produce shamanic states of altered consciousness based on high-voltage slow-wave hypersynchrony originating from the hippocampal-septal area.

Further studies of such mechanisms are needed to give a clearer understanding of shamanic altered states of consciousness and the psychological mechanisms of healing that are produced.

### Spiritualism

The broad term "**spiritualist**" is applied to one who believes that spirits of the dead can communicate with living persons. Persons known as "**mediums**" are felt to have special powers and a sensitivity to receive such messages. These persons are descendents in the hierarchy of the ancient primitive shamans who were always believed to be a link between the living and the spirits of deceased ancestors.

A **seance** is a session held by a medium in which he/she makes contact with the spirits. It is usually held in a darkened room in which participants sit around a table which may suddenly tilt or move. The medium may suggest that all present hold hands, thereby implying that the seance is honest with no trickery. However, the medium's feet are always free to produce the necessary movements. Hidden accomplices can also assist in the chicanery. Strange sounds occur, weird voices may speak through trumpets, and luminous bits of painted gauze float in the air, supposedly representing **ectoplasm** from departed spirits.

The spiritualistic movement surfaced in the USA at Hydesville, New York, in 1848 (8). It started with the innocent pranks of two little girls, the Fox sisters, who produced strange knockings on the floor over their mother's bedroom by bouncing apples tied to strings. Their mother interpreted these sounds as a haunting by the spirit of a peddler previously murdered in their farmhouse. An older sister purposely, and the mother unintentionally, implied that this disembodied spirit had taken possession of the children. Neighbors came to hear the strange sounds. Prominent Rochester Quaker abolitionists investigated the mystery and decided it was not a fraud. The children were frightened of exposure of their little trick and soon developed more sophisticated methods of deception. Newspapers became interested, and with the public's ever-present gullibility and interest in such mysteries, the word spread far and wide. Ultimately, the Fox sisters became celebrities and, managed by their clever and ambitious older sister, toured the country giving demonstrations of their spiritualistic abilities. Their methods became increasingly sophisticated and they drew large crowds wherever they went. It was a lucrative business until 1888, when the Fox sisters voluntarily made public the whole story of their 40 years of deception.

Too late, the damage had been done! The public had a large appetite for such deception, and enthusiasm for spiritualism spread rapidly in the 1850's and 1860's. Additional impetus came from the Civil War, as large numbers of relatives hoped to communicate with their lost sons and husbands (9). In the late 19th and early 20th Centuries, many spiritualistic mediums entered the field, and some became very famous. The Boston medium Margie was the wife of the physician Leroy Cranston, a lecturer at Harvard Medical School. She gave seances in her fashionable Beacon Hill home. Her husband was one of her dupes who believed in and supported her work until she was exposed by the famous magician Houdini.

Harry Houdini was born in 1874. He toured the world as a famous magician and escape artist. A major part of his later career was devoted to exposing fraudulent mediums. Although he hoped to prove that there was some truth in spiritualism, he never found it. He offered $10,000 to anyone whose methods he could not duplicate by common trickery. No one ever successfully claimed his offer and he exposed hundreds as charlatans. Large audiences came to his public demonstrations, which exposed the methods of fake mediums. After his death in 1926, his work was carried on by the "Great Dunninger," and other magician/mentalists who demonstrated and exposed methods of mind-reading on the stage, radio, and television (10,11,12).

Houdini was a friend, but also an antagonist, of Sir Conan Doyle, the famous English mystery writer, a leader in the spiritualist movement in England. Despite denial, Doyle always believed that Houdini somehow had supernatural powers. Houdini died on All Souls Day in 1926. On that day for the following 15 years, groups of mediums gathered in an attempt to receive a message from his spirit. That secret message, known only to his widow Beatrice, never came.

Similar booms in the spirit medium racket have been seen following World Wars I and II and the Vietnam and Korean conflicts, when bereaved relatives sought out mediums and fortune tellers in the hope of contacting their lost relatives. The advent of the wireless telegraph and later the discovery of roentgen rays in the 1890's sparked the belief that there might indeed be some sort of "celestial wireless," by which telepathic communication could occur not only with the dead but also between persons living at a distance from each other. A currently popular example is the belief in the effectiveness of absent prayer, in which the person sending the prayer believes that God will take time from his/her busy schedule to heed and take the action demanded by the praying person.

Belief in spiritualism, mental telepathy, and absent prayer continues unabated despite their fantastic nature and lack of serious scientific support. Albert Einstein professed skepticism about such *psi* phenomena since, according to the laws of physics, all known forces weaken with distance. Such is not the case with claimed telepathic experiences.

**Parapsychology**

The beginning of the new science of experimental psychology occurred during the early days of the spiritualistic movement, and there was confusion between the terms "psychological" and "psychical." The latter began to acquire a specific association with mental telepathy and spiritual phenomena, especially after the founding in England of the Society for Psychical Research in 1882. The American Society for Psychical Research was founded in 1884. William James, G. Stanley Hall, Joseph Jastrow, and other early leaders in American psychology were among the founders of this society. As laboratory investigations failed to reveal any scientific basis for the claims of spirit mediums, all the professors save one — William James — renounced any association with The American Society for Psychical Research. Major university departments of psychology moved away from research in spiritualism and instead focused on studies of the psychology of perception, belief, and religion (13).

The term "**parapsychology**" became applied to *psi* research. Grants for the study of parapsychology continue to be given to universities. Investigations include **psychokinesis**, the power to affect physical happenings through thought alone, including healing by absent prayer. The term "**extrasensory perception**" (ESP) includes not only **telepathy** (communication between humans and spirits and humans at a distance), but also **clairvoyance** and **precognition**, which come under the broad heading of prophecy or fortune telling. More recent areas of investigation include **near death experiences** (NDE) and **out of body experiences** (OBE), which are described as though one were travelling in a tunnel, seeing a person garbed in white, or having all of one's past life pass before the eyes. While these occurrences are usually presented as evidence for an afterlife, possible explanations include the physiological and biochemical changes seen with the depletion of oxygen to the brain that occur at the time of near-death occurrences. Such physiological alterations can also accompany extreme anxiety (14). Similar too are stories of **reincarnation, astral projections,** and abductions by strangers travelling in **unidentified flying objects** (UFO's). It is relevant that these latter types of observations have become popular only with the widespread interest and knowledge about space exploration. A probable explanation places them in the category of illusions and hypnagogic hallucinations (15).

The first major bequest given for the study of *psi* phenomena, or, as it was then called, "spiritualism," was in 1906 to Clark University in Rhode Island. Professor G. Stanley Hall was embarrassed by this gift, as he had little belief in spirits. Major grants for parapsychology were given to both Harvard and Stanford in 1913. Early studies there were performed on mediums to determine if they were frauds or naifs. Nothing definitive came of such research. Munsterberg at Harvard studied the famous medium Beulah Miller, who had been the subject of numerous investigations. He concluded that some persons such as she had "supernormal sensitivities," including the ability to read minute muscle movements of a person concentrating on test cards. If the subject was hidden from view, such "mind reading ability" failed.

In later studies at Duke University, J.B. Rhine, a botanist turned parapsychologist, carried on investigations of ESP using sophisticated controls and statistical methods. Again, as with all attempts, there were no solid supportive findings pertaining to the nature of clairvoyance. However, it appeared that some persons seemed to be able to beat the statistical averages. Martin Gardner (16) reviewed Rhine's work and concluded that there was ample room for human error here as well as in other telepathic phenomena. One could well include studies of absent prayer and, in the words of J.G. Pratt, conclude that ESP stands for "error some place."

It appears that there is no one explanation for the different kinds of *psi* phenomenon, nor has any acceptable proof of a scientific mechanism to support these claims been demonstrated. On the other hand, no number of negative results can prove the non-existence of *psi*, for there is always the outside hope that some new technique may someday come along to prove its existence. It is upon this sort of hope that much of the hype for New Age healing is built. Although many genuine and well-meaning persons are convinced that they can communicate by telepathy, find water by dowsing, or experience episodes of clairvoyance, no one can do these under conditions that rule out normal sensory information. People with a will to believe are easily duped into belief in the supernatural by reason of their own natural limitations in attention and sensory information, or are possessed of a strong desire such as a wish to communicate with deceased loved ones (17).

Ever-present charlatans seek to take advantage of the credulous. Uri Geller, an Israeli magician who began his career as an entertainer in Israeli night spots, toured Europe and the United States claiming supernatural powers. He demonstrated his expertise at psychokinesis by seeming to bend keys by mere thought. He fooled a group of Stanford parapsychologists, but was later defrocked by magicians. His methods have been exposed as fraudulent. Thus, even university parapsychology laboratories are in danger of fraud. The parapsychology laboratory at Washington University in St. Louis, established by a grant from the McDonnell Douglas Foundation, has not been immune to trickery despite scientific safeguards. After two years of studies of their psychokinetic abilities, a group of student volunteers finally confessed their plot, which deceived the investigator by practiced trickery.

In 1966, a group of Stanford University faculty, including physicists and psychologists with an interest in *psi* phenomena, founded the Parapsychology Research Group. A summary of their work and reflections after 25 years has been published in a silver anniversary book (18). They concluded only that much has been learned and that there is a need to incorporate *psi* into a spiritual, transpersonal model of the universe. They agree only on what they term "the probable existence" of telepathic phenomena.

## Divination

An important aspect of mysticism that has persisted through the ages is that of divination, the forecasting or prophesying of future events sometimes known as **precognition** (19). The priests of primitive religions practiced the sacrifice of animals on the altar. By examining the animals' entrails, the temple priests would tell of future events. Sacrifice of the lamb was a means of prophecy in early Judaism. It was thought that the shiny surface of the liver could provide a clairvoyant (clear-vision) picture of coming events. Among some Arabic tribes, the shiny surface of the fingernail, and among European cultures, the crystal ball and the magic mirror have served the same purpose for fortune tellers who would seem to find illusions of the future within their reflections.

Books of the Old Testament are filled with the proclamations of prophets whose pronouncements, after being told and retold, are today widely accepted by adherents of Protestant, Catholic, and Jewish religions. Various interpretations of such prophecies have led to heretic behavior and the formation of numerous dissenting religious sects. Muslims, too, believe that the word of God tells of the coming of the end of the world, a time when the dead will arise and all will be judged to experience either the joys of heaven or the punishments of hell. Every century has had its doomsayers who predict the date of the end of the world. These sects keep resetting the date when the event fails to occur.

No mention of prophets would be complete without the name of Nostradamus (20). This 16th Century French physician, herbalist, philosopher, and astronomer/astrologer was widely acclaimed, and was hired to advise the wealthy and prominent of his time. His predictions were written in ten books called the *Centuries*, each having 100 verses. These were written in the form of quatrains but were in no particular order. Composed in archaic Latinized French, their very obscure language has allowed many to read much into them. Even today, they are interpreted as prophetic of current world events. Various authors have written about Nostradamus, some of whom claim to have visited this famous prophet while under hypnosis, or who have suggested that they are his reincarnation. His prophecy of the end of the world — supposedly by the end of this century — has been the inspiration for nearly a half-hundred movies and videos. He was a forerunner of modern soothsayers such as the Edgar Cayces and Jeanne Dixons of our time.

In early China, divination was commonly used to forecast the outcome of wars and other important events. The emperor would summon his wizards (*wu*) to court. Two commonly used methods were **scapulomancy** and **milfoil lots.** The former was an interpretation of cracks made by heating the carapace of a tortoise or the shoulder bone (scapula) of a deer. In another method, the dried stalks of the Siberian milfoil plant were broken into short and long pieces, shaken together in a receptacle and poured onto the table. Patterns of the cracks in the bone or of the long and short sticks were presumably the origin of the designs of broken and unbroken lines that form the basis of the trigrams and hexagrams of ancient Taoism and shamanic beliefs. These designs make up the prognosticating patterns described in the *I Ching* (*The Book of Changes*), a popular book of fortune-telling found in every bookstore in the U.S.

**Tarot** is another popular method of fortune telling (21). Tarot is the French name for procedures involving a deck of 78 cards used for games and for fortune-telling. The cards are divided into four major suits: cups, swords, wands, and pentacles, within which there are 22 major trump cards: fool, magician, high priestess, empress, emperor, hierophant, lovers, chariot, strength, hermit, wheel of fortune, justice, hanged man, death, temperance, devil, tower, star, moon, sun, judgment, and world. These are pictures of the things, people, events, ideas, and emotions that populate and shape the imagination. Variations of these cards, beautifully decorated, are used to inspire the imagination of the viewer, whose visions are then interpreted as descriptions of past or future events. Not only is Tarot a means of fortune-telling, but since its inception in the 15th century, it has inspired poets, artists, and authors and has served as a vehicle for many occult and arcane organizations throughout history.

Although fortune tellers and psychic counselors use such methods as tarot cards, tea leaves, and palm reading, none is as universally popular as **astrology**. This was practiced by the Chaldaean priests of Babylon hundreds of years B.C.E. Even at that time, a distinction was made between astrology and astronomy, the latter being attempts at a scientific understanding of the universe. The early Greeks held a general belief in prophecy and predestination. A religion that added interpretation to the signs of the sky was well received, so magical astrology blossomed and was even taught along with medicine on Hippocrate's island of Cos.

The mysteries of the heavens and of any possible magical effect they may have on humans is a universal preoccupation. Thus, with some cultural differences, astrology also flourished in early China and India. Astrological signs were important to the early alchemists and the witches of the early Middle Ages. In addition to ordinary horoscopes, decumbency charts which foretold the outcome of an individual's disease were widely used in the Middle Ages. At that time, with a rise in printing, astrological almanacs became popular among the common people. Royalty had their own astrologers, and Popes John II and Clement VIII were reputedly adept at astrology.

With the rise of scientific investigation in the 17th and 18th Centuries came a clear separation between astronomy and the magical pseudoscience of astrology. Yet today, belief in astrology seems stronger than ever. Persons of modern historical importance, including Hitler and President Reagan, have depended upon astrological prognostications. Recent tabulations indicate that there are 10,000 practicing astrologers in the United States. One thousand of these practice full-time. Americans spend 200 million dollars a year on astrology. Omitting the space program, this is more than twice the amount that is spent on astronomical research. Twenty percent of people believe in astrology and millions read the horoscopes that appear in more than 1000 daily newspapers, only some of which carry disclaimers that these daily forecasts are "for entertainment purposes only." Tabulations of predictions made by astrologers are less than 10% correct, far less than by chance alone. People forget the misses and remember only the rare hits.

It is interesting that whereas the astrological Zodiac contains only 12 constellations, others have been discovered by astronomers. This has affected every one of the Zodiac signs. Also the precession of the equinox over the last several centuries has further eroded traditional astrological beliefs. To quote the London Times, "Astrology is pure foolishness. Not even their signs correspond to the truth (22)."

Why all of this interest in prophecy? The current turning to astrology is perhaps a desperate groping for some miraculous solution to the increasing turmoil and grave problems facing individuals in today's world (23).

**Mystical Healing**

Miraculous healings have long fascinated humans. They are commonly interpreted as occurring by the direct intervention of a supernatural being in the course of an otherwise fatal illness. Whatever unusual behavior preceded the cure is, from association, often given credit for the "miraculous recovery," whether it was prayer, an herb, a change in lifestyle, or the laying on of hands. Although the media and T.V. make much of these rare occurrences, modern medicine interprets them as spontaneous healings, possibly action of the body's immune system.

For the many miracles that color the stories of Biblical times and have been credited to powers of the Essenes or other healing priests, modern psychology has another answer. The commonly recognized psychological mechanisms of suggestion and dissociation give a natural explanation for these stories of miracles attributed to saints, shrines and relics handed down in legends from pre-Biblical times through the Middle Ages. Lack of scientific facts to otherwise explain disease conditions and common natural phenomena set the stage for widespread belief in magical and supernatural causation of illness and healing. Cases of sudden recovery from blindness, deafness, and paralysis, now recognized to be of probable common hysterical origin, were fertile grounds for reports of miraculous healings. A religious healer often had to prove him/her self by the performance of miracles, justifying the claim of supernatural powers leading to deification.

Modern miracle healings of hysterical paralysis are accomplished readily by hypnosis. With the advance of scientific knowledge, cases of "grand hysteria" have become increasingly rare in psychiatric clinics in the United States. I have, however, accomplished such relief of symptoms on several occasions during my practice of psychiatry. My most recent experience was the sudden healing of hemiplegia in an hysterical woman from a remote rural area of Turkey. This was during a demonstration of hypnosis at a medical school in Istanbul. It stands out in my memory, for due to the language barrier, the cure was accomplished with the aid of an interpreter.

In the United States at the turn of the Century, there were many reports of healing by the laying on of hands. Chiropractic medicine (*cheiro*, hand, and *practikus*, to do, from the Greek) was founded by a magnetic healer who cured a case of hysterical deafness by mysteriously manipulating the neck of his patient. The power of healing by touch, so prevalent in Biblical times, has come down through the ages as a method commonly used by evangelical revivalists in their "faith healing" ceremonies in which their hands presumably act as a conduit of healing power from God. One recent T.V. evangelistic healer asked his naive viewers to place their hands on the screens of their home television sets in order to receive the healing powers that he would send to them by satellite.

In China, the external *Qi Gong* healer acts in similar fashion, sending power from his hands to heal and influence the behavior of patients. Studies of *Qi Gong* reveal changes in the brain similar to those reported in EEG studies of hypnosis. In a recent article, Wu Xianghong (24) describes the rise of interest in the paranormal in China. He cites the exposure of hoaxes and failed research attempts along with rampant superstition and lack of critical training in science as explanations of the *Qi Gong* phenomena.

In alternative medicine, other techniques of healing power from the hands go under such names as Reiki, Rosecrucian healing, and most recently, Therapeutic Touch, a debatable procedure taught by nursing professor Delores Krieger.

Interestingly, such power emanating from the hands was claimed by Mesmer, one of the early founders of hypnotism. Following his custom, some stage hypnotists today seek to amplify their power of suggestion with dramatic hand gestures. Strange behaviors seen at both stage demonstrations of hypnosis and evangelical religious healings include falling, appearing to faint, and unusual body mannerisms. These are simply the behaviors and emotions aroused by suggestion in susceptible individuals who come to the stage or altar at the invitation of the hypnotist or the evangelist's call to "come forward and be saved."

Army psychiatrists in World War I observed that hysterical symptoms occurred more frequently among common and less educated soldiers than among officers recruited from the ranks of persons with more education. This parallels the observation that cures by magical means are commonly seen in primitive and developing countries where scientific knowledge is not widely distributed to the population.

**Body Energies**

The term "body energy" is widely used in discussions of alternative healing. Phrases like "to increase body energy," "to balance body energy," "to release energy blocks," or "to increase energy by detoxification" imply that this is a known biological force than can be manipulated for healing. In actuality, there is no such force. "Body energy" is a metaphysical term based on philosophical and religious concepts. It is often used synonymously with "life force," which has an etymological relationship with "spirit" and "soul," terms for universal debate. Perhaps we should go along with the French Philosopher Bergson whose *elan vitale* simply implies that body energy represents the possibility for independent action of a human during that period of living between birth and death.

Energetic concepts derived from primitive cosmological and anatomical beliefs vary from culture to culture and have changed with the progression of biological and physical knowledge. In Ayurvedic medicine, it is *prana,* the mysterious energy that travels up the column of *chakras*. In Traditional Chinese Medicine, the concept of "energetic medicine" centers about *ch'i (Ch'hi, Qi, Xi)* , which comes in various forms — "blood *ch'i*," "breath *ch'i*," etc. — and travels about the body in hypothetical "*meridian* channels." An ancient Taoist belief is that life comes about as a combination of the male (*Yang*) and female (*Yin*) *chi's*. With the increased popularity of Traditional Chinese Medicine in the West and the scramble by naive promoters of various methods of holistic healing, alterations in *ch'i* have been widely accepted as the explanation for various healing effects.

In the West, dating from the first century C.E. when Galen's anatomical dissections seemed to demonstrate that nerves were hollow structures, it was believed that pulsations of the brain, pumping fluid through the nerves, energized movement of the muscles. This "hydraulic theory" came to an end in the 17th Century when Munro demonstrated that nerves were not hollow.

In early theologies and in Christian Science and other healing religions of today, it is believed that the energetic **power of God** is channeled through the healing minister. This was the power demonstrated by Jesus, the Essenes, and other Biblical healers.

In the shamanic healing of North American Indian tribes, the power of the **Great Spirit** passes into and energizes the medicine man healers. **Reflexologists** hold that there is a mystic body energy that travels from points on the sole of the foot to each body organ over hypothetical channels that have never been demonstrated anatomically. For **auriculotherapists**, there is the similar concept of energy travelling from the ear. The mysterious energy that is supposed to occur with Chinese external *Qi Gong* was demonstrated on television during a recent show on Alternative Medicine by Bill Moyer. This same type of *Qi Gong* energy failed to occur under the experimental conditions designed by researchers of CISCOP, the Committee For Scientific Investigation of Claims of the Paranormal (25). That such old hypotheses about healing through manipulation of "body energies" are gaining acceptance today is evidence of the universal belief in magical forces.

**Breathing** was designated by ancients as the important energy giving life force. They viewed with awe those independent functions of the human body that began at birth with the first breath and ceased at death with the last breath. From such observations, life appeared to be solely dependent upon breath. A story in the Judeo-Christian Bible states, "And the Lord formed man of the dust of the ground and breathed into his nostrils the breath of life: and man became a living soul." A similar statement is found in the *Koran*. Both ancient Chinese medicine and Ayurvedic medicine give special attention to breath as a factor in the life forces, called respectively *ch'i* and *prana*. The Greek word *pneuma* and the Latin *spiritus* also include in their meaning both breath and life spirit.

**Auras** are reportedly seen about the bodies of healers and in the halos of angels. These purportedly indicate a mystical type of energy. The ethereal corona of light is said to be intensified around the hands when healing is taking place. The aura around a person who is ill is said to be of a different color and character. Kirlian photography, an image made upon a photographic plate when the body is subjected to an electronic charge, is believed by some to represent an image of the aura. Scientific explanations derived from laboratory investigations of this phenomenon have robbed it of its own mystical and romantic "aura" (26).

Such healing energies are believed by some to have a cosmic origin. The Ancient Greeks explained the energy of a lightening storm to be the anger of Jove. In China, when heaven and earth were thought to be out of balance, the *yin and yang* of individuals were also out of balance and illnesses prevailed. As late as 1890, the Chinese had soldiers fire volleys from their muskets to frighten away the demons of the plague. Wilhelm Reich promoted various types of "orgone" collecting devices to accumulate healing forces from the heavens. Religious tales about spiritual and mystical healings are believed by many to be factual rather than allegorical. Belief in their reality exists, despite an increasing body of scientific knowledge regarding the physical makeup of the world that could be used to give a different interpretation to such mysteries.

*Quantum physics* is touted by some as an explanation of the basis of "body energy" healing. Viewed in the light of today's knowledge, the world around us appears as three-dimensional matter only because of the way our sense organs perceive it. The electro-magnetic spectrum is a broad one and we sense only a very small part of it. Some animals can hear or see beyond the abilities of humans. Perhaps then, the argument goes, some persons may fall at extreme ends of the bell curve of the normal distribution of sensory abilities. These persons could then be the gifted "healers" who claim to perceive energies that others do not. That a few persons could have abilities not possessed by the majority is in no way, however, evidence of any universal importance of such healing abilities.

Perhaps the psychic healer who emanates "energy" from the hands has a looser molecular and electron structure on the surface of the body than other persons. All "normals" are expressed as a median from the extremes. We all lie at different locations under the bell-shaped Gaussian curve. When the healer rubs the hands together to "charge" them (as is often the custom), even more electrons might be "pried loose." Pertinent to this concept is the work from Elmer Green's group (27), which found that when electronically isolated and measured carefully, Non Contact Therapeutic Touch (NCTT) healers could, by their "mental intention to heal," generate a measurable voltage larger than that of non-NCTT control subjects. Whether this voltage, extremely small as compared to the far more powerful currents used in electroacupuncture or TENS units, has the potential to produce any measurable healing effect on the body has yet to be convincingly demonstrated. Certainly, the caring and stroking of one person by another can induce a person's feelings of warmth and love, a process that might stir an individual's immunologic responses for healing, whether it is a "placebo" or psycho-neuro-immunologic mechanism. The nursing profession represents *par excellence* a caring profession, and hence, there is a strong attraction for nurses to attend classes teaching "therapeutic touch," a procedure which certainly emphasizes their ability to project an atmosphere of loving care. In the Middle Ages, it was the king's touch that was described as emitting a similar healing energy. This healing energy was supposedly transferred to coins engraved with a likeness of the king. These were called "touchpieces."

Although humans cannot see or hear some vibrations unaided, we have developed scientific instruments that signal what is happening in the range of ultra-sonics, telecommunications, and the infra-red areas of the spectrum. Our knowledge of these forces tells us much about the world. What we ordinarily perceive as material is in reality largely space, containing matter made up of small groups of molecules, which are in turn made up of atoms, which are in turn composed of minute universes of electrical charges — electrons and quarks. We cannot, unaided, see this electronic latticework which appears to us as solid. How solid is well demonstrated by the opposition one feels when trying to move a metal object through a strong electromagnetic field. It is as though you have come against a solid wall. Were our eyes so attuned, we would see that the whole world — all that surrounds us, including our bodies — is composed primarily of empty space occupied by miniature whirling electrical galaxies. This, then, is the ultimate real "body energy" that lies at the basis of all living matter. Perhaps in time, as we explore the molecular make-up of the human body, we will ultimately learn to deal with such forces. Today, however, holistic healers do not have any scientific knowledge about the manipulation of such forces that is not available to scientific medicine.

*Biological energies.* We are only now beginning to understand the role of the molecules of second messenger systems and calcium channels. Cell membranes are permeable to the molecules of medicines that set in motion various cell energies catalyzed by enzymatic action. These are the actions occurring within our solid-appearing body organs. Once that sackful of chemical substances called the human body is set in motion by receiving its first breath of air, it continues to be "alive," pre-programmed by DNA, its master architect, for its whole lifetime. The body is composed of a symbiotic collection of organs and physiologically interacting systems. It continues to live, powered by enzymatically controlled chemical reactions, until some outside accident or the DNA program itself no longer orchestrates the continual enzymatic changes that are necessary for the chemical processes of life. At this point death occurs.

Recent studies of the processes of cell death ("apoptosis") have shed new light on human mortality. Although some cells of the body can clone, or replicate themselves by a process of division known as meiosis, this process has its limits. The replication of hair cells, for example, goes on at a much faster rate than the replacement of liver cells. All cells, however, appear to have a limit to the number of generations possible for their kind. Apoptosis is the mechanism in the genes that stops cell duplication after a set number. Thus, aging and ultimately, death of the human body occurs when the cells of essential organs are no longer able to repair cell death. The search for the "fountain of youth," the ability to live indefinitely, will not be found in the waters of Florida as Ponce de Leon believed, but rather in the laboratories of microbiologists.

*Nervous energy*. For centuries, people believed that life stopped when breathing stopped. With the development of the electro-encephalograph early in this century, it became possible to see the electrical activity of the brain. It was found that the cells of the brain, the organ of central body control, continues to function as long as oxygen and blood are supplied mechanically. Final or "brain death" occurs when the brain cells no longer show any evidence of producing electrical energy.

Cognitive thought and memory in humans involves the left cerebral cortex, the hippocampus and amygdala. These are areas situated above those brain stem centers that are responsible for automatic actions such as respiration and the beating of the heart. The EEG delineates from brain activity three states of mind: waking, sleeping, and dreaming. A look at these sleep mechanisms reveals yet another, more scientific way to view the body energy concept.

Usually as daylight turns to darkness, a shift occurs away from the daytime discernible high level of energy that is characterized by alertness, muscle activity, sensory responsiveness, and vocalization. Sleep, on the other hand, is a state of observed quiescence. These two phases, waking and sleeping, are controlled by two different brain areas and body chemicals. Waking and action are aminergic (serotonin and norepinepherine); sleep and dreaming are under cholinergic control. The shift is governed by a circadian clock *(zeitgeber)* the supra-chiasmic nucleus (CSN) of the ventral hypothalamus. Melatonin from the pineal body plays a role here. When the circadian shift occurs, this CSN clock turns off and a nucleus in the pontine brain stem turns on the cholinergic mechanisms.

Sleep is characterized by five stages with distinct EEG patterns. Early in sleep, the subject normally descends quickly through lighter stages and enters stage IV, or deep sleep. This lasts for several hours and is followed by a series of interruptions known as REM periods, first described in 1957 (28). They occur 6-8 times per night, lasting up to 90 minutes each. In REM, although the body is resting and cannot move, the brain is active, vital functions continue, and the eyeballs move rapidly. The mind is filled with the contents of the dream material supplied from the brain's memory stores. Recent studies seem to point out that this aimless pouring over the contents of memories stored in circuits in the brain's 100 billion neurons is what restores and keeps memories alive. Thus, REM becomes important for a continuous updating of our memories. Apart from memory storage, sleep states are essential for the presence and strength of the processes of homeostasis. Thermoregulation and immune function are maintained by REM sleep.

Despite much religious and philosophical theorizing, there is no single static executive center like Descarte's pineal "seat of the soul." Rather, the higher life center for memory and observation of behavior is to be found in this essential network of neurons and nuclei of the brain that are in constant flux. We can anatomically distinguish between those parts and functions of the brain responsible for maintaining the chemical processes of life, the brain stem, and those more forward areas which perform the executive functions responsible for the higher life functions of living. It is here that neuroscientists place consciousness, an evanescent, ever-changing evaluation of the self.

Dissociation of motor and sensory functions from conscious awareness can occur and are readily seen in hypnosis and hysteria. Hilgard (29) speaks of a "hidden observer" as that part of the pain nervous system that produces physiological reactions to a nociceptive impulse, while the hypnotized person consciously denies feeling any pain sensation. Crawford (30), using brain-mapping techniques, localizes this "supervisory and attentional control system" to an area in the far frontal cortex.

The subconscious, non-volitional brain, orchestrates the communication of the various systems of our body, which "talk to each other" by sending out molecules that fit into specific receptor sites of the cells receiving the message. This fit of key into lock unleashes the chemical reactions basic to life. This is the mind/body relationship that today is being studied within the speciality of neuro-psychoimmunology. On another scale of organic life, when chemicals cross the synaptic space between neurons, they initiate electrical depolarization processes along nerve axons that can induce muscle fibers to move limbs.

Even a thought is a neuro-electrical event occurring within the structure of the brain. In his famous experiment on a conscious patient, neurosurgeon Wilder Penfield (31) could find with electrical stimulation of nervous tissue only those points on the brain which produced visible consciously recognized movements. Now, with our advanced recording procedures, we can even see the electrical disturbance in brain tissue when a thought occurs — the intention to move — just milliseconds before the actual movement occurs. With the measuring devices we now have, we cannot yet find in any material substance the conscious will that makes that decision. Hence, we posit free will as an unknown or spiritual entity. As Candice Pert (32) has shown, to think is to create a brain chemical event, to create a messenger molecule. In fact, as long as the body is alive, it is in constant conversation with itself. Awake, asleep, and dreaming, the organs of our body "talk to each other" in this chemical manner.

These taken all together then are the physiologically determined manifestations of the energetic life force — marvelous yes, but magical? No!

## Conclusion

What then is "life energy" but simply those rather homogenous electronic particles of which all matter is composed? Thought is the interaction of some of these electronic forces. In specific combinations, molecules make up the organs and systems of the human body. These organs and systems interact molecularly. Individual cells, acted upon by enzymes, follow their predetermined patterns of function, and this is the body energy of life. Claims about healing produced by manipulating "body energy" have nothing to do with imaginary *chakras* or *meridians*, but everything to do with how the mind can influence the body. Strong belief excites known mechanisms of interaction that can heal the body through an effect upon hormones and the nervous system. Promoters of New Age medicine claim that such mind/body medicine was imported by them from the Far East. In reality, mind/body medicine, under the title psychosomatic medicine, has been taught in U.S. medical schools since early in this century.

Many explanations of alternative medical procedures are not matters of fact, but beliefs based on observations of body function made in pre-scientific days. For alternative healing techniques to be acceptable to allopathic practitioners, they must undergo the same rigorous double-blind controlled evaluations that the FDA requires of new drugs. This has not been done with most of these healing methods.

From the viewpoint of the individual holistic healer, there is only one correct technique. That is the one which he/she believes and practices. Many such healers are without medical training and hence, unschooled in the critical thinking of scientific medicine. They are prone to accept at face value observations and testimonies that are made without factual verification.

And so we can conclude that there is a body energy. But it is energy at a subatomic level that exists within and is substantiated by Einstein's theory and the findings of experiments in the physics laboratory. It is not a mysterious force that flows like a stream of water through hypothetical *meridians* or a fancied *chakra* column. This kind of body energy obeys the laws of physics, not the caprice of magical thinking. The direction of placement of an acupuncture needle does not stem or reverse the flow of "*meridian* energy." Neither meditation nor the manner of breathing can hasten "*chakra* energy transportation." However, for the believer, such manipulations can produce a strong placebo effect.

A factual approach to understanding the existence of body energy at the atomic and molecular level opens the door to a useful interpretation of observations about these mysterious energies that have puzzled humankind for centuries prior to the advent of scientific medicine. It is the forces within and between molecules that we must manipulate to enhance healing. This is done by supplying substances that the body requires to manufacture the enzymes and chemicals that sustain the chemical reactions of the life force; food, medication, herbs and vitamins. These enzymatic and biochemical reactions can also be effected by various mechanical manipulations that impinge upon the nervous system, producing local electron perturbations that, while moving only infinitesimally, initiate conductances in the central nervous system that are so amplified as to produce resultant meaningful and distant effects. These can be produced by supplying external energies through the chemicals of neuro-pharmaceutical agents. Externally applied energy by means of neuroelectric acupuncture has been shown by Han to release specific neuropeptides, endorphins, enkephalins, or dynorphins at specific frequencies of stimulation. Pert has suggested that such acupuncture may release as many as 70 different neuropeptides. Mental manipulations — imagery, meditation, hypnosis, exercise, and some types of biofeedback — induce bodily changes through the release of specific biochemicals such as neuropeptides and hormones. These can effect a variety of body organs and systems. This is also the basis of the placebo effect. Theories of psycho-neuro-immunology thus explain the power of a strong belief in the shaman's arcane rituals.

The magical concept of a mysterious "body energy" has no place in modern medicine. Only the application of the laws of physics and the scientific techniques of physiological and biochemical investigations will determine which medical treatments, allopathic or alternative, can best maintain the homeostatic functioning of the human body.

## REFERENCES

1. Sagan, C. (1996). *The demon-haunted world: Science as a candle in the dark.* New York: Random House.
2. Romano, C. (1994). The art of deception or the magical affinity between conjuring and art. *The Linking Ring, 74,* 59-65.
3. Houdin, R. (1959). *Memoirs of Robert Houdin.* Philadelphia: Evans.
4. Blumberg, D., et al. The physician and unconventional medicine. *Alternative Therapies, 1*(3), 31-35.
5. Davis, W. (1985). *The serpent and the rainbow.* New York: Warner Books.
6. Stearn, J. (1968). *Edgar Cayce, the sleeping prophet.* New York: Bantam Books.
7. Wright, P. (1995). The interconneactivity of mind, brain, and behavior in altered states of consciousness: Focus on shaminism. *Alternative Therapies, 1*(3), 50-56.
8. Hull, B. (1977). *The billion dollar bait.* Deland, FL: Volcanda

9. Brown, E. (1983). Neurology and spiritualism in the 1870's. *Bulletin of the History of Medicine, 57,* 563-577.
10. Christopher, M. (1975). *The illustrated history of magic.* New York: Thomas Crowell.
11. Dunninger, J. (1974). *Dunninger's monument to magic.* Secaucus, NJ: Lyle Stuart.
12. Booth, J. (1984). *Psychic paradoxes.* Los Alamitos, CA: Ridgeway Press.
13. Coon, D. (1992). Testing the limits of sense and science: American experimental psychologists combat spiritualism. *Amer Psychol, 47,* 141-151.
14. Blackmore, S. (1987). The elusive open mind: Ten years of negative research in parapsychology. *Skeptical Inquirer, 11,* 244-255.
15. Blackmore, S. (1992). Near death experiences: In or out of the body? *Skeptical Inquirer, 16,* 34-45.
16. Gardner, M. (1981). *Science: good, bad, and bogus.* Buffalo, NY: Prometheus Books.
17. Grey, W. (1994). Philosophy and the paranormal: Part 1: The problem of "psi." *Skeptical Inquirer, 18,* 149.
18. Kane, B.; Millay, J.; & Brown, D. (1993). *Silver threads: 25 years of parapsychology research.* Westport, CT: Praeger.
19. Rawcliffe, D. (1959). *Illusions and delusions of the supernatural and the occult.* New York: Dover Publications.
20. McCann, L. (1984). *Nostradamus: The man who saw through time.* New York: Greenwich House.
21. Giles, C. (1992). *The Tarot: history, mystery and love.* New York: Simon & Schuster.
22. Gamez, A. (1995). Zodiac crashes down. *Skeptical Briefs, 5* (2), 1-2.
23. Culver, R., & Ianna, P. (1988). *Astrology: true or false?* Buffalo, NY: Prometheus Books.
24. Wu Xianghong. (1995). Paranormal in China. *Skeptical Briefs, 5,* 1-3, 14.
25. Kurtz, P. (1988). Testing psi claims in China: Visit by a CISCOP delegation. *Skeptical Inquirer, 12,* 364-376.

26. Watkins, A., & Bickel, W. (1986). A study of the Kirlian photography effect. *Skeptical Inquirer, 10*, 244-257.
27. Greene, E., & Greene, A. (1986). Biofeedback and states of consciousness. In B. Wolman and M. Ullman (Eds.), *Handbook of states of consciousness.* New York: Van Nostrand Reinhold.
28. Kleitman, N. (1962). *Sleep and wakefulness.* Chicago: University Chicago Press.
29. Hilgard, E., & Hilgard, J. (1975). *Hypnosis in the relief of pain.* Palo Alto, CA:William Kaufman.
30. Crawford, H., & Gruzelier, J. (1992).*Midstream view of the neuropsychophysiology of hypnosis: Recent research and future directions in contemporary hypnosis research.* New York: Guilford Press.
31. Penfield, W. (1976). *The Mystery of the mind.* Princeton: Princeton University Press.
32. Pert, C., & Snyder, S. (1973). Opiate receptors: demonstration in nervous tissue. *Science, 179*, 1011-1014.

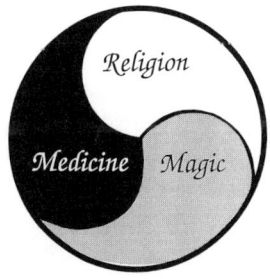

# III

## PLACEBO — THE POWER OF "I BELIEVE"

I RECALL as a small boy that a doctor in our town dispensed a wondrous tonic. It gleamed with an iridescent golden glow, its vapor penetrated to the top of one's head, its taste was most foul, and if one could tolerate it in the mouth, it burned all the way down. Taken in the spring, it prevented illness, cured the widest variety of afflictions, and when rubbed on the skin, could banish warts. Indeed, it was the magic cure that worked miracles, approaching those of the healers of ancient days that I had learned about in Sunday school.

One summer in later years when I was home from medical school and eager to sit at the feet of our town's wise old family doctor, he told me the secret of this powerful medicine — sulfur, molasses, black pepper, and a wisp of camphor. This was my very first knowledge of placebo medicine.

Later, as a house officer in a large county hospital, I learned that only rarely did the new breed of scientifically trained doctors use a placebo intentionally and only then in a manner suggestive of scorn and derision. When some patient's complaints caused an overworked physician to awake in the small hours of the night, he would use "placebo" as a dirty word. Upset by the intrusion on his all too brief sleep, he might instruct the nurse to "quiet" the patient with a sugar pill or "sterile water hypo."

A number of years passed before I became fully acquainted with a third facet of placebo medicine. As a professor and medical researcher, I found the placebo had a respected place in evaluating the effectiveness of newly discovered drugs in controlled studies.

Viewed from any vantage point, the placebo is certainly a kind of magic. In keeping with the dictionary definition of a miracle as "any wonderful or amazing thing," the placebo produces miracles on demand and does so in a way that appears unexplainable.

Through the centuries, history has recorded recoveries that were not explained by known scientific means. Such cures were often attributed to the intervention of some supernatural power, and persons responsible for invoking the cure were deemed "magicians," or even "saints." It is now known that in the hands of most healers, modern as well as ancient, the placebo can produce such miracles. It can cure disease, although in itself has no known scientific reason for such cure, and it requires only the unspoken incantation of both physician and patient ... "I believe."

The long, dark years preceding the 19th Century were times when physicians had little to offer their patients other than hope, support, and magic rituals. These, with the patient's faith and trust, formed placebo medicine. The administration of cupping, purging, plasters, and cathartics, added little to the curative effect and may well have impeded the body's natural healing powers. Excessive bleeding by his physicians may well have hastened the death of President George Washington. Today, we are so accustomed to thinking of medicine in scientific terms that we forget that for thousands of years patients were cured by witch doctors and shamans who possessed not even a shred of scientific medical knowledge.

Slowly, with many observations, the gathering of data, and the advent of the scientific method, procedures and drugs with specific actions came into being. Some plants had been observed to have a healing action, but these were mostly crude mixtures. In China in the year 1000 A.D., a pharmacopoeia of over 1,000 substances existed, crude herbs often mixed with animal artifacts. Such herbs are purified, their active principles extracted and used for the treatment of specific illnesses. Using the chemical structure of these drugs as a model, new drugs have been designed and synthesized that are even more effective in treatment. But even these drugs do not work for everybody and at all times. Often when a new drug is introduced with much fanfare, it seems powerfully potent. With repeated use, the drug seems less potent and finally may be discarded entirely. A common saying about new drugs is "use them while they still work."

This phenomenon perplexed physicians and sorely troubled the pharmaceutical industry. By the 1950's, the placebo was recognized as an important part of healing and a serious power to be dealt with. To ensure patient safety, increasing emphasis was placed upon clinical trials of new drugs. The Federal Drug Administration (FDA) is concerned not only that new preparations have a low incidence of side effects, but also that they should have some specific biological benefit beyond what could be seen with a placebo.

Thus, double-blind experiments became the order of the day. In this procedure, two groups of volunteer patients, all with the same disease, were randomly assigned and studied. One group was given capsules of the new drug to be tested. The other group was given "look-alike" capsules containing some inert substance — "sugar pills." Neither the doctor giving the pills nor the patients receiving them knew which were which, hence the term "double-blind." Only at the end of the experiment were the capsules identified. The amount of benefit that occurred with the "sugar pills" was called the "placebo effect." If the degree of relief seen with the new substance was no greater than that which occurred with the inert substance, the new drug was shown to be without any therapeutic value. The use of such double-blind procedures has proved to be of value in preventing the promotion and sale of many worthless drugs.

Thus, the Random Clinical Trial (RCT) became the basis for measuring treatment effectiveness in Allopathic Medicine. A key ingredient of the RCT was placebo effect. In holistic medicine, the placebo effect is too often all there is. The efficacy of such treatments may be judged on a naturally occurring improvement in the patient's condition coinciding with the administration of some herbal preparation. Thus, the clinical observation or verbal report of a treatment's therapeutic result was formerly the only standard of care to be achieved. Now the "gold standard" in scientific medicine is treatment outcome minus the placebo effect. We are thus able to obtain some measure of the importance of physician/patient interaction.

Beecher (1) pointed out that total drug effect is its active effect plus its placebo effect. In his example, if 75% of patients gain relief from post-operative pain by a large dose of morphine, one third of this relief is judged to be placebo effect. In one report, "A standard dose of morphine given to placebo-negative persons was effective in 54%, whereas the same dosage given to placebo-positive individuals was effective in 95%."(2)

Placebos provide an effect just as "real" as that of the drug they mimic. The stronger the drug, the stronger the placebo. It has been shown that the more intense the pain, the greater the placebo response; that is, the greater the patient's need for help, the better the effect of the placebo (3). Although most commonly, placebo effect is related to control of pain, it can have many other effects on the body. Placebos affect both the organs and their autonomic functions. Pupils change size, and the pulse and blood pressure rise or lower. One study of placebo versus Metamucil for the treatment of irritable bowel syndrome demonstrated placebo's power to calm intestinal peristalsis (4).

Placebos can have an ameliorating effect on coughs and colds (5), seasickness and peptic ulcer (6), allergic conditions including status asthmaticus (7), hay fever (8), rheumatoid arthritis (9), hypertension (10,11), angina pectoris (12,13,14), headache (1, 15), mental depression (7,16), vasomotoric disturbances, claudication intermittens (17), and others.

A dramatic study of placebo surgery was a comparison of the effect of mammary artery ligation, a procedure that was popular in the mid-1950's for the treatment of angina pectoris. This operation was based on the assumption that such ligation would improve the blood flow to the heart, and success rates of 65%-75% were reported. Although unacceptable by today's ethical standards, two studies were reported of sham operations in which only an incision was made in the chest wall and resutured without any further surgery. In one report, all the non-ligated patients and 76% of those with ligation experienced an increased exercise tolerance and less need for nitro-glycerin (18).

Placebos can also produce side-effects. Beecher's study (1) reported: drymouth, nausea, sensation of heaviness, headache, difficulty concentrating, drowsiness, relaxation, fatigue, and sleep. Wolf and Pinsky (19) reported weakness, palpitation, nausea, rashes, epigastric pain, watery diarrhea, urticaria, and angioneurotic edema of the lips. It should be noted that the physician's influence can also produce unfavorable results. These are termed "nocebo" effects. Beware the physician with a negative attitude!

Outside the field of licensed medical practice, placebo therapeutics, though often unrecognized as such, flourish. Many ancient healing practices originating in primitive, pre-scientific times have been dredged from the past. They are described as working in some mysterious fashion and are promoted to the public under such umbrella terms as "holistic" and "alternative." When therapists with no medical training use such methods to treat patients with psychosomatic conditions, the strong placebo component may at times be even more effective in producing an amelioration of symptoms than less dramatic scientific medical treatments.

The importance of the placebo became ever clearer to me as over the years I watched physicians practice their healings. Doctors differ greatly in the "art of medicine" and the quality of their bedside manner. Patients, too, come in many varieties. Some seem optimistic and heal quickly; others are dour and pessimistic and heal slowly or not at all. I learned that people get well for many reasons, not all of them explained by drugs or surgery.

One manner of healing occupied most of my time during four years in medical school. That was the promotion of recovery through the administration of specific drugs and treatments for specific illnesses which affected specific organ systems. Thus, it was "penicillin for pneumonia," "aspirin for a fever," and hundreds of other curative formulae targeted at carefully diagnosed diseases. It was not until later when I specialized in psychiatry that I became fully aware of the powerful effect of the doctor/patient relationship and its effect on results obtained in the giving of prescription drugs.

Non-specific mind/body methods of treatment are currently not sufficiently stressed in the curricula of Allopathic medical schools. Such methods, however, are the basic fare of alternative healers. Both types of healers, however, take advantage of the body's own healing mechanisms aided by the "tincture of time." Both types of healers recognize that vitamins, diet, and exercise are important as preventive measures and as aids in strengthening the body's resistance to disease. Both types of healers rely in part on the placebo response without ever giving it full recognition for the role it plays in the treatments they offer.

There has been much speculation about how placebos work. One commonly accepted theory is that placebos relieve anxiety. Certainly, anxiety increases the subjective severity of any illness. It is well known that anxiety turns up the volume control on pain perception. Relief of anxiety can diminish the severity of pain and, as clearly demonstrated in wounded soldiers during World War II by Beecher, placebos do just that.

Studies of the personality of placebo responders have yielded equivocal results. Some have shown them to be outgoing, verbally and socially skilled, enthusiastic, and generally well-adjusted persons. Placebo non-responders, on the other hand, have been characterized as being belligerent and antagonistic toward authority. Lasagna and co-workers (2) reported that regular church-goers showed a higher percentage of placebo positive persons than non-churchgoers.

Levine (20) demonstrated that naloxone blocked the placebo effect. This he interpreted to mean that endogenous opioids were responsible for the placebo response. Later studies (21,22,23) confirmed this observation, including one report of cross-tolerance between the placebo effect and morphine. Despite some criticism, the evidence in support of a neuropeptide hypothesis to explain the placebo response appears strong. Mihic and Binkert (24), for example, who reported no reversal of the placebo effect by naloxone, used a model of ischemic pain which is relatively insensitive to this opioid antagonist (25).

The analgesia associated with fear, as well as the symptoms of panic and phobic anxiety, are transmitted through the nor-adrenergic system, and hence render a poor placebo response. It becomes clear that the opioid-serotonergic pain-inhibiting system which is activated by neuro-electric acupuncture, TENS, and physical activity is also activated by psychological mechanisms such as placebo action.

The widespread nature of the placebo response can be explained by the origin of not only B-endorphins, but also adrenocorticotropic hormone (ACTH) and the alpha, beta, and gamma variants of melanocyte-stimulating hormones, all from the common precursor pro-opiomelanocortin (25,26,27,28). This complex molecule is found mainly in the nucleus arcuatus of the ventro-medial part of the hypothalamus, which projects to the limbic structures, septum, and amygdala for emotional control, the periventricular and periaqueductal grey matter for pain control, and the nucleus tractus solatarious which controls cardiovascular reflexes (29). Placebo responses should therefore be manifest in situations where these hormones exert their activity. Of particular importance, then, are stressful situations with accompanying anxiety (30,31,32) where the placebo can participate in a balancing of homeostasis, including both anti-inflammatory and immunosupressive effects (33). This explains early observations that placebo can increase adrenocortical activity (34) and reduce serum lipoproteins (35).

Positive thinking, the expectancy of cure, the belief, or, as the Bible says (Matthew 21:21), the "faith of a grain of mustard seed" produces the placebo miracle. One study showed that 25% of patients felt better once they had called their physician for an appointment. And fully 50% "felt better" while sitting in the doctor's waiting room. I have had patients who came to my office for the first time say, "I don't know if it's the weather or not, but my pain is not as severe today as it was yesterday." The white coat can invoke the suggestion for healing. Too often, physicians forget what magic lies in the staff of Aesculapius. The more strongly the physician believes in the curative strength of what he is doing or giving, the greater will be its effect.

Some patients demand that the doctor give them pills. They feel the physician has not treated them properly unless they leave the office with a prescription in hand. It is, therefore, up to the physician to use his wisdom in deciding whether the situation justifies placebo medicine. As Dr. Murray Jarvik, Professor of Psychiatry and Pharmacology at the UCLA School of Medicine in Los Angeles said, "It is clearly not malpractice to prescribe ineffective medicine so long as it provides a certain degree of psychological support for the patient and as long as it does not interfere with a truly effective treatment (36)."

We can thus conclude that the placebo does have the power of any and all types of drugs and treatments. It is not something to be ignored, despised, or neglected. Rather, the placebo should be recognized for what it is, a powerful ally of the healing profession. It should be accepted, employed and used to enhance and amplify the effect of whatever is being done on the patient's behalf. On the other hand, it should not be forgotten that in the hands of charlatans, pure placebo medicine may be employed primarily to lighten the contents of the wallet rather than the burden of discomfort.

## REFERENCES
1. Beecher, H.K. (1955). The powerful placebo. *JAMA, 159*, 1602-1604.
2. Lasagna, L., et al. (1954). A study of the placebo response. *Am J Med, 16*, 770-779.
3. Wolk, S. (1959). The pharmacology of placebos. *Pharmacol Rev, 11*, 689-704.

4. Longstreth, G., et al. (1981). Psyllium therapy in irritable bowel syndrome: A double-blind study. *Ann Int Med, 95*, 53-56.
5. Gravenstein, J.; Devloo, R.; & Beecher, J. (1954). Effect of antitussive agents on experimental and pathological cough in man. *J Appl Physiol, 7*, 119-139.
6. Backman, H.; Kalliola, H.; & Ostling, G. (1960). Placebo effect in peptic ulcer and other gastroduodenal disorders. *Gastroenterologia, 94*, 11-20.
7. Wayne, E. (1956). Placebos. *Brit Med J, 2*, 157.
8. Baldwin, H. (1954). How to evaluate a new drug. *Am er J Med, 17*, 722-727.
9. Traut, E., & Passarelli, E. (1957). Placebos in the treatment of rheumatoid arthritis and other rheumatic conditions, *Ann Rheum Dis, 16*, 18-21.
10. Grenfell, R.; Briggs. A.; & Holland, W. (1963). Antihypertensive drugs evaluated in a controlled double-blind study. *South Med J, 56*, 1410-1416.
11. Shapiro, A. (1956). Consideration of multiple variables in evaluation of hypertensive drugs. *JAMA, 160*, 30-39.
12. Amsterdam, E.; Wolfson, S.; & Gorlin, R. (1969). New aspects of the placebo response in angina pectoris. *Amer J Cardiol, 24*, 305-306.
13. Benson, H., & McCallie, D. (1979). Angina pectoris and the placebo effect. *New Eng J Med, 300*, 1424-1429.
14. Evans, W., & Hoyle, C. (1933). The comparative value of drugs used in the continuous treatment of angina pectoris. *QJ Med, 2*, 311-338.
15. Dowson, S.; Lewith, G.; & Machin, D. (1985). The effects of acupuncture versus placebo in the treatment of headache. *Pain, 21*, 35-42.
16. Hollister, L., et al. (1967). Drug treatment of depression. Amitriptyline, perphenazine, and their combination in different syndromes. *Arch Gen Psychiatry, 17*, 486-493.
17. Bounemeaux, H., et al. (1985). Placebo-controlled, double-blind, two-center trial of ketanserin in intermittent claudication. *Lancet, 2*, 1268-1271.

18. Brody, H., & Yates, A. (1990). The placebo response. In D. Wedding (Ed.), *Behavioral medicine*. St. Louis: C.V. Mosby.
19. Wolf, S., & Pinsky, R. (1954). Effects of placebo administration and occurrence of toxic reactions. *JAMA, 155*, 339-341.
20. Levine, K.; Gordon, N.; & Fields, H. (1978). The mechanisms of placebo analgesia. *Lancet, 2*, 654-657.
21. Fields, H., & Levine, K. (1984, August). Placebo analgesia – a role for endorphins. *TINS, 7*, 271-273.
22. Grevert, P.; Albert, L.; & Goldstein, A. (1983). Partial antagonism of placebo analgesia by naloxone. *Pain, 16* (2),129-143.
23. Hargreaves, K.; Dionne, R.; & Mueller, G. (1984). Pituitary beta-endorphin release and subjective responses to surgical stress following naloxone, fentanyl or placebo in humans. *Pain, (suppl 2)*S406.
24. Mihic, D., & Binkert, E. (1978). Is placebo analgesia mediated by endorphin? *Abstracts, Second World Congress on Pain, Montreal, 1,*19.
25. Kaada, B. (1982). Neurophysiological mechanisms of pain suppression and cutaneous vasodilation induced by transcutaneous nerve stimulation (TNS) and acupuncture—a review. (*Legevitenskap og livsvisdom, 'Festschrift* to Tollak B. Sirnes on his 60th anniversary, October 17, 1982). Bergen: University Press.
26. Chretien, M., et al. (1979). From B-lipotropin to B-endorphin and "pro-opiomelanocortin." *Can J Biochem, 57*, 111-121.
27. Loh, Y., & Loriaux, L. (1982). Adrenocorticotropic hormone, B-lipotropin, and endorphin-released peptides in health and disease. *JAMA, 247*, 1033-1034.
28. Swaab, D., et al. (1981). The distribution of MSH and ACTH in the rat and human brain and its relation to pituitary stores. In *Endogenous peptides and learning and memory processes* J.I. Martinez, et al. (Eds.). New York: Academic Press.
29. Nieuwenhuys, R. (1985). *Chemoarchitecture of the brain*. Berlin: Springer-Verlag.
30. Szara, S. (1982). Opiate receptors and endogenous opiates: Panorama of opiate research. *Prog Neuropsychopharmacol Biol Psychiatry, 6*, 3-15.

31. Akil, H. et al. Stress induced increases in endogenous opiate peptides: Concurrent analgesia and its partial reversal by naloxone. In H.W. Kosterlitz (Ed.), *Opiates and endogenous opioid peptides*. Amsterdam: Elsevier.
32. DeWied, D., & Jolles, J. (1982). Neuropeptides derived from pro-opio-cortin: Behavioural, psychological and neurochemical effects. *Physiol Rev, 62*, 976-1057.
33. Guillemin, R.(1978). Peptides in the brain: The new endocrinology of the neuron. *Science, 202*, 390-402.
34. Cleghorn, R., et al. (1950). Anxiety states: Their response to ACTH and to isotonic saline. *Proc First Clin ACTH Conf,* Philadelphia: Blakiston.
35. Rinzler, S., et al. (1953). Effect of heparin in effort angina. *Amer J Med, 14*, 438-447.
36. Jarvik, M., & Schneider, N. (1984). Degree of addiction and effectiveness of nicotine gum therapy for smoking. *Amer J Psychiat, 141*, 790-791.

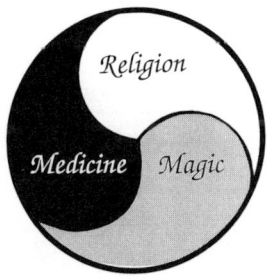

# IV

# HEALING BY FAITH
## RELIGION IS GOOD FOR YOUR HEALTH

*"If there were not a God,
it would have been necessary to invent one."*

*Voltaire*

HEALING is a natural phenomenon, a built-in power responsible for maintaining life against hordes of microbial invaders and scores of mishaps. The body's own recuperative powers which ensure the existence of humans have been with us from the beginning. Only in the last 100 years, however, has scientific medicine developed rational means to successfully destroy parasitic, bacterial, and viral pathogens and to surgically remove tumorous growths and repair body defects. Such actions assist the body's own healing powers. Prior to this century, people got well not because of what was done *for* them, but in spite of what was done *to* them. Cautery, cupping, bleeding, purging, and the spells of witches and charlatans did little to aid the healing process. Rather, it was the patient's belief in the treatment, the placebo effect of faith, that assisted in his or her recovery. Seeking help from the relics of saints and praying at holy shrines were *par excellence* the model of healing by faith. Studies have shown that persons who are intrinsically religious have better health and healing than those lacking such faith. Research has scientifically supported the premise that the mind can significantly affect the body's health. For not only must the placebo effect be counted seriously into the equation of healing, but the whole new science of psychoimmunology has added incontrovertible evidence that attitude and emotion affect healing directly through strengthening the function of the immune system.

While the above might seem disconcerting for those who believe that only God creates healing miracles, it need not be so. This is no victory for science over religion. How the facts are interpreted depends upon the individual's own belief system. For the believer, The Great Creator of all things created all scientific knowledge as well.

## Historical

From the very dawn of civilization, magic, medicine, and religion have been intrinsically intertwined. Described as the first physician to appear in the mists of antiquity, Imhotep was a priest, astrologer, healer, and minister to King Zoser (2682-2613 B.C.E.). After his death, he was revered as a deity in the great triad of gods at Memphis. Here in the temple, patients prayed and slept, believing that methods of cure would be revealed in their dreams. An ancient Egyptian papyrus reads, "He who treats the sick must be expert in magic, learned in the proper incantations, and know how to make amulets to control disease." Today, priests perform more humble duties. It is only in the Eucharist that the clergy take part in a routine, though invisible miracle — the transformation of wine and bread into blood and flesh.

Ancient religions of Greece and Mesopotamia were polytheistic. The pantheon of Gods contained those who were good and those who were malevolent. The latter could cause disease, the former prevent or cure illness. Early Assyrian tablets denote methods for curing illness by driving out demons. In the famous healing temples of Aescelapius in Greece, religious methods of healing were employed.

In China, 3000 B.C.E., the physician/acupuncturist was a bird-like superhuman creature. In France, drawings on the wall of a cave around 20,000 B.C.E. show an animal-like creature, the healing priest. In the *Pali Canon* of Buddhism, the Sakyamuni Buddha was a great healer. One of the most sublimely beautiful art works in the whole world is his replica in an attractive man-made grotto high on a mountain top in the valley of the Silla Kings near Kyongju, South Korea.

About 500 B.C.E., Zarathustra, founder of the Zoroastrian religion, taught that prayer would bring divine intervention and the cure of illness. Similar was the emphasis by the early Hebrews on health and healing (Exodus 15:26) when Moses revealed that God promised, "I am the Lord that healeth thee." All of the early prophets were healers (Psalms 103:3).

"Bless the Lord ...who healeth all thy diseases." It was within this Judaic culture that Jesus Christ demonstrated a healing power amply described in the New Testament. The commission given by Jesus to his Apostles was to "heal the sick."

The *Qur'an*, holy book of Muhammadanism, holds itself as "...a guidance and a healing for those who believe." Islamic healers of both Sunni and Shia persuasions had elaborate theological formulae for curing illness. In all of these, prayer played a most important part.

The term "faith healing" is a broad one, including any phenomenon in which a physical disease is cured by any means other than drugs, surgery, or a recognized form of manipulation or psychological treatment. It is a field lying somewhere between medicine and religion. If it worked as well as some faith healers say, it would be the greatest means of lowering the cost of medical care available. However, proof is lacking. English physician Louis Rose (1) spent 20 years trying — but failing — to document even one case of what he considered a *bona fide* "miracle" cure. A British Medical Association's committee in 1956 reported on "divine healing." (2) They found "...no evidence that there is any type of illness cured by 'spiritual healing' alone which could not have been cured by medical treatment." Their report stated that "the evidence suggests that many such cases which claimed to be cured are likely to be either instances of wrong diagnosis, wrong prognosis, remission, or spontaneous cure."

In Western thought, the outstanding healer was Jesus of Nazareth. One verse in every seven of the Gospels, and one in fourteen of Acts refers to the type of therapeutic activity that led John the Baptist to conclude that here was more than just another "magus" representing a cult such as that of the Essene healer priests. It was only after his death, however, that Jesus was recognized as no ordinary man but as the Christ or Messiah. And in the four Gospels, some fifty paranormal events, many of these healings, are attributed to Jesus.

Christ's techniques for healing were prayers, the laying on of hands, and commands for the sufferer to pursue certain courses of action. After his death, his healing powers became legendary. The disciples had received the command to "heal the sick, cleanse the lepers, raise the dead, and cast out devils." (Matthew X:8); or, as in Mark XVI:16, "lay hands on the sick: and they shall recover."

Today we find such traditions of healing in churches throughout the world and in all of the major religions. Some have separated teaching and preaching as a congregation-related function and have relegated the healing ministries to church-related hospitals. In this fashion, most non-profit hospitals in America were started by and remain loosely associated with major religious groups.

In the early centuries of Christianity, faith healing remained a major therapy. Through the 4th Century and into the time of St. Augustine, the Roman Catholic Church had many healing saints. In Catholic Christian theology, priests were given healing powers through rites of ordination. Any failure to heal was regarded as evidence of sin on the part of the healer. Such priestly power to heal by prayer could remain after death in the sacred relics or at the shrines of such priests who after death were designated as saints.

Through the 7th Century, these ritually produced paranormal cures were regularly reported. However, after the Council of Nicaea in 325 C.E., the philosophy of the Church began to change as it assumed a dominance over Western thought. This dominance was to endure for 1000 years. The church became more formal and organized, revelation was considered complete, and there was a return to the fatalism of the old covenant which regarded all phenomena, including disease, as immediate expressions of God's will. In accordance with the doctrine of original sin, mankind was doomed to "innocent" suffering. Pain was to be borne patiently and efforts were to be concentrated on preparing the soul for salvation.

Monastery hospitals such as St. Albans (800 C.E.) were founded as a revival of physical medicine was beginning. Such institutions, however, were mostly infirmaries preparing for a peaceful sanctified death rather than true treatment. The Sacrament of Extreme Unction, anointing the dying patient with holy oil, was important. Exorcism became increasingly common because it was believed that most diseases were due to actions of the Devil. The situation degenerated as priests began to add to their income by selling cures, a scandal which led to condemnation by the Lateran Council of 1123 C.E.

Around the 12th Century, Jews of the later Rabbinical period and the followers of Muhammad began to make progress in orthodox healing; hence, the beginnings of medicine existed alongside saintly cures. When, however, neither physician nor priest could help, patients turned to the village "leech," barber, apothecary, witch, or wise-woman. The witches provided most of the healing in medieval Europe. Cupping, bleeding, sweating, and primitive surgery were also practiced by barber surgeons. The list of healing practices included the use of talismans, neolithic sites, interventions by elves and fairies, holy groves, healing wells, relics of violent death, moon-magic, excreta, and herbs. These practices bore little relation to the Gospel tradition of healing. There was a continuing belief that diseases were caused by malevolent spirits. Witchcraft was prominent in the 15th through 18th Centuries. The Inquisition was established in the 13th Century to punish all heretics against Catholicism. Many of its victims were witches, mostly women, and they numbered in the thousands.

The belief that the King was to some degree a priest was a tradition that spread from the East in Graeco-Roman times. King Olaf of Iceland, Clovis the first Christian King of France, St. Louis of France, and others were believed to have the power to heal. The King's healing blessing could even be confirmed by coins ("touchpieces"), which bore his likeness. Healing by the King's touch reached a peak in 1686, when on an Easter Sunday, King Louis XIV of France ministered to a crowd of sixteen hundred.

An even stronger force for healing was astrology, which, from its origin in Egypt (about 500 B.C.E.), spread through Rome, bringing with it a belief in Pythagorean number magic and the Aristotelian theory of elements. This blended with the primitive medical thought of the times and gave its name to the chemicals and metals used in healing. In the 16th Century, astrology became the dominant force in medical healing.

For the centuries spanning the Reformation and the counter-Reformation, the Catholic healing shrines began to lose some appeal. The rise of the new Protestant groups under Luther and Calvin placed greater emphasis on the belief that sickness was God's pre-ordained punishment for original sin. Martin Luther believed that for those who had strong faith, no disease was incurable.

Also living at this time were persons for whom religious creeds were only incidental. Their challenge was to heal pragmatically. The first of the documented post-Reformation healers to be found in Commonwealth Britain was Valantine Greatrakes. He was an Irish Puritan known as the "stroker." He stroked patients with his hands and asked God "out of His abundant mercy" to heal them. As his reputation grew, he began to hold healing clinics, during which he would "squeeze" the ailment to an extremity and then out of the body. Before the fading of his powers in 1667, shiploads of people from London crossed the Irish Sea to be healed by his ministrations.

A century later, an ordained priest of the Roman Church, Father Gassner, used a shortened form of exorcism of his own invention instead of the official bell, book, and candle. In keeping with his belief in demonic possession, he would order the demon within the patient to reproduce the symptoms of an epileptic fit. Every month, he treated some two thousand sufferers of all persuasions and is said to have achieved immediate symptomatic relief for many of them.

Another priestly healer was the Reverend Prince von Hohenlohe, born in Wurtemberg in 1794. He was noted for his emphasis on "absent healing." His most famous case was the dramatic healing of a novice nun living in Chelmsford, Massachusetts. She suffered from an infection of her arm, which was swollen to a diameter of 15 inches. Hohenlohe prayed for her from Bamberg, Germany, thousands of miles away, and "overnight her arm healed, the swelling diminishing to a five inch circumference."

There has been a recent revival of interest in the possibility of "absent prayer." (3) Great emphasis has been given an experiment carried out at San Francisco General Hospital, in which 393 patients with heart disease were subjects of a double-blind prayer experiment. Patients were randomly assigned to two groups. One group was prayed for, the other was not. While the results showed that those prayed for fared better than the "control" group, there are many possible errors in the study (4). Other clinical studies are less dramatic, and it would require many more careful scientific studies to prove any healing power of directed absent prayer. No lesser figure than Albert Einstein has questioned the mechanism of such telepathic events on the grounds that they are counter to the known principle in physics that the greater the distance, the weaker the signal. Even "brain waves," the demonstrable microvolt electrical emanations from the brain, require powerful amplifiers to detect them with electrodes placed directly on the scalp. Dossey (3) calls mind/body medicine

"Medical Era II" and speaks of "Era III" as the future in which all types of distant healing will be possible, including intercessory prayer and various telesomatic events. This, he says, will be possible because "mind" is unbounded and infinite in space and time. Support for such beliefs come from observations in quantum physics which claim that once sub-atomic particles have been in contact with each other, they "always retain that contact" regardless of the separating distance. Dossey states, however, that "so far no one has been able to demonstrate that cancer or any other disease will predictably disappear by using prayer, meditation, or any psychological or spiritual method whatever."

Healing by hypnosis, which had its early roots in Egypt, became prominent in the mid-1700's and was promoted by Franz Anton Mesmer, a Viennese physician and astrologer. He promulgated the idea that his healing powers were due to an "animal magnetism" emanating from his hands.

Others followed in Mesmer's footsteps. James Graham, a Scot, built a grandiose "Temple of Health" in London. In addition to "electrical and other scientific appurtenances," he featured a "Grand Celestial Bed." He was one of the first to realize the financial potential of sexual anxiety, and rented out the bed to childless couples for 500 guineas a night.

Before the middle of the last century, there was a revival of Jewish faith healing in the form of the Hasidic movement. At this time, a more rational growth of medicine was occurring in the Arab world. At the same time, however, in the United States—particularly in New York and New England—centers for varieties of unconventional healing arose. These were often associated with esoteric philosophies and new religious sects. In Rhode Island, a "Doctor" Newton is said to have treated over a quarter of a million subjects with a healing derived from traditional Christian beliefs of love and prayer, abetted by hypnotism, electro-magnetic devices, and manipulation. He developed a "hydropathic cure," in which he poured scalding water over his subjects.

An itinerant healer and hypnotist, Phineas Parkhurst Quimby was a founder of the Swedenborgian "New Thought" movement in New England. One of his successful patients was the 41-year-old Mary A. Morse Baker Glover Patterson Eddy, then in the throes of her second unhappy marriage. Where all orthodox medical methods had failed to relieve her numerous symptoms, Quimby succeeded. She, an unsophisticated housewife, became his devoted follower. When he died, she took over his methods and established the healing sect called Christian Science (5). She described the system as one of her own origination and published the (since then much revised) *Science and Health with Key to the Scriptures*. Herein she claimed that all illnesses are only "false beliefs." She regarded herself as the supreme healer. She preached that cures could only be achieved within her own discipline and that any failure to achieve a cure was due to skepticism on the patient's part. Christian Science now has thousands of specially licensed, fee-charging nurses and practitioners.

Hundreds of sects and groups of people and individuals today believe in spiritual healing. Most demonstrate their ability to heal while alive, but some, characteristic of the ancient Roman Catholic healers, demonstrate an increased healing power at their gravesides after death. One in particular, an Arab monk, Charbel Makhlouf, claimed comparatively few cures before his death in 1898, but in 1950 his grave in Lebanon became a popular healing shrine for both Moslems and Christians. A century after its founding, the shrine at Lourdes, France, continues to attract thousands of suffering patients from all over the world.

With the speeded tempo of life and the advent of radio and television, healers of all types have become increasingly visible. Harry Edwards in England, Billy Graham, Oral Roberts, the Bakers, and many others in the United States are representative of this group. Healing is done by prayer, the laying on of hands, and even ancient exorcism rituals. Television evangelists heal by means of "absent prayer."

The potential financial profit of modern day evangelism is tremendous and thus the temptation for charlatanism, fraud, and abuse is great. Before his death, the Reverend Jim Jones, messianic leader of a cult of abuse, demonstrated his ability to cure cancer and raise the dead. After his death, persons came forward, stating that they were threatened by Jones and were paid to fake death and illness. Such cults of abuse are all too common and create great suffering and even death among their followers (6).

The desire to see favorable results where none exist is the basis upon which suggestive cures can be developed. However, to date, no systematic studies have proven scientifically any remarkable results of such evangelistic healing methods. Only anecdotal claims exist.

## Modern Healing

Chiribin (1992), in his discussion of *Healing and Spirituality* (7), points out that each of the three agencies for healing — medicine, psychology, and religion — directs its focus respectively to a different part of human existence — body, mind and soul. Hippocrates introduced the concept of holistic medicine in 400 B.C.E. and treated the whole man. Somehow, during the Middle Ages, the attitude toward healing changed, with treatment of the physical body becoming the prerogative of the medical profession, while care of the mental and spiritual aspects became the sovereign right of the church.

During the 19th and 20th Centuries, medicine became increasingly scientific and laboratory-oriented. Medicine was reductionistic and physicians looked primarily for the cause of the disease with little attention being paid to the person carrying the disease. Only recently has there been a re-emphasis on the total person with a revival of interest in the effect of the mind on the body's response to disease. Yet how important this is! The Center for Disease Control has shown that as many as 80% of patients have self-limiting disorders that are within the range of the body's healing powers.

Most people are aware that how they feel and think can affect illness. Petitional prayer, asking God's help for recovery from illness, is a common practice (3). The Gallop Poll taken in the U.S. in 1944 and repeated in 1981 found that 95% of the population believe in God. Sixty-six percent feel that religion is important and 72% give positive answers to the statement, "My whole life approach is based on my religion."

With religion so important to the bulk of the population, and with recognition of the significance of mental attitude upon disease, the power of spiritual commitment should receive greater recognition from physicians as a powerful ally in the treatment of their patients.

It is important for the physician to recognize that healing is a part of many different faiths (8). Although Christianity is the dominant religion in the United States with over 100 million followers, significant numbers of the other major world religions — Judaism, Islam, Hinduism and Buddhism — will be included among any patient population. Within the Christian Church, over 250 separate groups with their own individual interpretations of the Bible, sacraments, and ways of worship exist.

Jesus Christ is viewed differently by different religions. Like Buddha and Mohammad, he is seen as one of the world's great holy men. For some he is, although outstanding, simply another Old Testament prophet. For most Christians, he is the true Son of God. To some but not all, he is of virgin birth, and for those accepting the Trinity, he is God Himself. Whatever the interpretation, however, viewed historically, the singular work of Jesus to a great extent involved healing, restoring, and making whole. Such love and caring, taught by the faith that carries his name, can significantly affect healing.

Christianity, however, has no monopoly on the healing power of such love and care. God is good and He/She spoke to all religions. It would appear then, that physicians — regardless of their beliefs — would utilize the healing power of the patient's religion. However, focused as they are upon the scientific and physical aspects of disease, physicians may tend to neglect the spiritual. Some even become apostate.

The profession of psychiatry, above all branches of medicine, should be the one to place value upon the spiritual aspect of human beings. Yet, of American Psychiatric Association members, only 39% profess to be religious. Henry, Sims and Spray (9) studied 3,147 psychotherapists and found that 29% — almost one third — had turned away from theistic beliefs. The highest number apostate were psychoanalysts: 40% compared with 26% for nonpsychoanalytic psychiatrists, clinical psychologists and psychiatric social workers.

Larson, a leading worker in this field (10), studied 3,777 articles that appeared in four leading psychiatric journals over a five-year period. He found that a religious measure was used in less than 3% of all quantitative studies. Only 1% of 2,348 studies paid any attention to religious variables. In only three studies was a religious measure a central variable of the study.

In the 15th Century, Melanthcon, an associate of Martin Luther, coined the word "psychology" from "psycho" (spirit or soul) and "logos" (word or thought). In early years, psychology focused on the study of the "soul." Later, with anatomical knowledge of the brain and its functions, psychologists studied the "mind." More recently, psychology has looked at the measurement and control of "behavior." As one wag put it, "Psychology first lost its soul, then its mind, and now is having trouble with behavior!"

Clark Hull, often thought of as the father of modern psychology in the U.S., taught and wrote frequently on the subject of religion. With psychology's current emphasis on treatment methods and on the relationship of physiological measures to behavior, psychology has for the most part given up studies of the psychology of religion. In undergraduate colleges today, the subject is rarely taught.

Times have thus greatly changed since Benjamin Rush (1745-1813), the "Father of American Psychiatry," stated: "A religion of some kind is as essential to the mind of man as air is to respiration." In the 20th Century, Sigmund Freud, by far the most influential figure in modern psychiatry, described himself as a "Godless Jew." In his book, *The Future of an Illusion,* he states, "Religious beliefs are illusions, fulfillments of the oldest, strongest and most urgent wishes of mankind." He attributes the origin of religious belief to early Oedipal conflicts in which the developing child sees God as a replacement of the father figure. Albert Ellis, the contemporary gadfly of psychiatry, has stated that religion is in many respects equivalent to irrational thinking and emotional disturbance. "The less religious," he said, "the more emotionally healthy."

**Studies of Religion and Health**

Larson and Larson (11) extensively reviewed the literature looking for evidence of a positive effect of religious belief on behavior, mental health, physical health and well being.

They found that the kinds of questions asked by various surveyors of the literature included: (a) Do you belong to a church? (b) Do you attend religious services? How frequently? (c) Apart from attending religious services, how important is religion to you (very, somewhat or not important)? (d) Do you pray? How? **Colloquial:** (ask God for guidance); **Petitional:** (ask God for help with events or material things); **Ritualistic:** (read prayer book); **Meditative:** (feel presence of God); **Intercessory:** (ask God to help others). Meditative and colloquial prayer are more indicative of a serious personal religious nature. The effectiveness of intercessory prayer, despite claims, remains an open question (12).

Most important is an **intrinsic religious commitment**, indicated by such statements as "my whole life is based upon my religion," "being born again," and "closeness to God." These are all measures of a positive religious commitment, as are feelings of existential well being, happiness, and spiritual satisfaction. The term **extrinsic religious commitment** refers to a lesser commitment to religion. It is indicated by the use of ritualistic and petition prayer and such comments as, "I go to church mainly because I enjoy seeing people I know" and, "What religion offers me most is comfort in times of trouble and sorrow."

The effect on health of confession, a practice long recognized by both Catholic and Protestant churches, may well relate to studies on the beneficial effects of prayer. Shamans, priests, and psychotherapists have all found that "opening up" has beneficial effects on the psyche. "Confession is good for the soul," is a common expression. Research has shown that confession has a beneficial effect on blood pressure, insomnia, psychological well being, and the immune system. If the confession involves one's deepest thoughts and emotions and is about sins not previously confessed, the attendance at health clinics is said to be decreased.

**Specific Areas of Study**

The Larsons (11) compiled a considerable amount of evidence from published literature supporting the belief that strong religious commitment can have a positive effect on both mental and physical health. Some of that evidence follows.

*Alcohol Abuse.* Alcoholics Anonymous (13) has long placed emphasis on turning responsibility for life over to a "higher power." It takes as a tenet of faith that compelling belief can improve mental health, aid in resisting temptation, and help organize life into what is and is not important. In studying the effects of the Alcoholics Anonymous movement on mental health, however, one must distinguish the effect of group support from that of individual belief.

Larson and Wilson (14) reported that persons who abuse alcohol rarely have strong religious commitment, while Gartner et al. (15) reported that six out of seven studies found that persons with higher levels of religious involvement are less likely to use or abuse alcohol.

*Suicide.* Comstock and Partridge (16) demonstrated that persons who do not attend church are four times more likely to commit suicide. Larson and Larson (11) quote two studies showing that the national decline in church attendance predicted higher nationwide suicide rates. Seven studies showed that religious persons have fewer suicidal impulses. This, they felt, relates to a higher level of self esteem.

*Drug Abuse.* The Larsons (11) found that drug abuse is related to the absence of religion in a person's life. In 11 of 12 studies, frequency of church attendance is more strongly related to drug abstinence than any other variable. The lowest percentage of substance abuse is found in conservative religious groups.

*Juvenile Delinquency.* Gartner et al. (15) pointed out that religious participation has consistently proven to be a deterrent to delinquency. Five of six studies reviewed by Argyle et al. (17) show that personal church attendance correlated negatively with delinquency.

*Divorce and Marital Satisfaction.* One of the most important predictors of marital stability is church attendance. Larson reviewed seven studies and found a positive relationship with religious commitment (regular church attendance) and self-reported marital satisfaction. He showed in a 1978 study that church attendance predicted marital satisfaction better than any of eight other variables. Tavris (18) found that very religious women report greater happiness and satisfaction with marital sexual adjustment than either moderately religious or non-religious women.

*Depression.* The Larsons (11) found four studies showing that a higher amount of religious commitment results in less depression. Gartner (15) reported a study on elderly women recovering from broken hips. Those with stronger religious beliefs and practices were less depressed and walked farther at time of discharge.

*General Well Being.* In their assessment of general well-being, the Larsons (11) found that persons who attend religious services regularly report lower levels of psychological distress than infrequent attenders and non-attenders. Six studies assessed religious states and psychological states at several periods over time. They reported an increase in psychological positive functioning following an increase in religious participation.

*Physical Health.* An elderly population living in the vicinity of New Haven, Connecticut, was followed for two years. Measured over time, the less religious had mortality rates occurring at twice the rate of the more religious.

An analysis in an 8- to 10-year follow-up of 2,700 persons found that women with increased church attendance have lower mortality rates. One study found that the risk of dying from arteriosclerotic heart disease is much less for men who attend church weekly. The risk is twice as high among infrequent church goers.

In the last 30 years, 20 studies were made on the effect of religious factors on blood pressure. In all but one study, certain religious commitment measures were associated with lower blood pressure or lower rates of hypertension.

Studies across different religious denominations revealed that especially highly devout, behaviorally strict groups such as Seventh Day Adventists and Mormons have significantly lower rates of hypertension-related morbidity and mortality than comparison populations. These groups follow health-producing behaviors as part of their religious commitment, including vegetarian diet and avoidance of alcohol, tobacco, and caffeine.

Levin and Vanderpool (19) studied the impact of religion on men's blood pressure and found that those with a high level of church attendance and who considered religion very important had a significantly lower diastolic blood pressure than those for whom religion was of little importance and who had a low record of church attendance. The average was a 5 mm difference in diastolic blood pressure. Studies show that a reduction of 2-4 mm can reduce cardiovascular disease by 10-20%.

Smokers who rated religion as very important were seven times less likely to have an abnormal diastolic blood pressure than smokers who gave a low rating for the personal importance of religion.

Levin and Schiller (20) surveyed 250 studies in epidemiological literature. They looked at nine health-related areas: cardiovascular disease, hypertension and stroke, colitis and enteritis, general health status, general mortality, cancer of the uterus and cervix, all other non-uterine cancers, morbidity and mortality in the clergy, and cancer in India. They found positive correlations between commitment and health. They concluded that "infrequent church attendance should be regarded as a consistent risk factor for morbidity and mortality."

Traditionally, it has been found that better-educated persons have better health. In these studies, it was found that higher religious commitment has as much impact on health as higher level of education.

David Spiegel of Stanford (21) studied 86 women with metastatic breast cancer. He reported a relationship between their belief systems and psychological adjustment to their illness. He described four types of belief system: **a)** a personal psychological belief system in which the patient's mental attitude, emotional state, and coping behavior are believed to play the central role in controlling and explaining the onset and course of cancer; **b)** a religious belief system in which prayer and faith in God both control and explain the cancer; **c)** a medical biotechnological belief system in which scientific explanations of causation and control are employed; and **d)** a fatalistic belief system in which chance and the arbitrary nature of the world are regarded as sufficient explanations of control and causal attributions. He found that those belief systems giving patients a greater perception of self-control over the course of the illness were predictive of less mood disturbance and greater improvement.

**Possible Physiological Basis of this Health-Producing Phenomenon**

Faith has been described as a blend of conviction and imagination. Primitive persons were convinced that the shaman or witch doctor would help them recover from their illness. Incantations and colorful healing ceremonies and rituals were fertile material for the imagination. The individual with a culturally determined conviction that "God helps" may readily transfer this faith to God's emissary, the faith healer.

In the field of psychiatry where the psychological aspects of healing are maximized, no evidence exists that one school of psychotherapy is more effective than any other, for it is the attitude rather than the theory that is important.

Physicians have long known that an ability to inspire expectant trust in a patient has something to do with the success of treatment. This is the basis of the placebo response, which, in addition to any biochemical or other action of a medical treatment, causes a physiological healing response triggered by the emotional reaction of the patient.

When patients have faith in the doctor and in the treatment being given, that strong belief elicits a placebo response. As Beecher (22) demonstrated in the 1950's, the placebo response adds strength to whatever treatment is being given. The physician's strong belief that the treatment will be effective may be communicated to the patient verbally and also non-verbally by an air of confidence.

For thousands of years, patients were cured mainly at shrines and by a variety of witches, charlatans, and folk healers. An example of the continuing healing power of shrines is that of Lourdes, France (23). Here at 12:30 p.m. on February 11, 1850, an illiterate, asthmatic, 14-year-old girl, Bernadette Soubirous, began seeing visions of the Virgin Mary. She was later canonized as St. Bernadette. In the years following her visions, great claims of healing have been made by those who bathe in the spring waters of the Shrine at Lourdes or pray to Saint Bernadette. The healings here have been much analyzed. Important factors in these phenomena are: the anticipatory expectancy of preparing for the long journey (the shrine fails to heal those who live close by); the reinforcement of faith from the streams of returning pilgrims with their testimonials; the physical impact of the icy waters; and the emotional appeal of the religious ritual. All of these suggest powerful psychological mechanisms for the healings that occur.

Belief in the power of prayer, "faith of a grain of mustard seed" (Matthew 17:20) has given support to healing by religious suggestion. This is dramatically seen at Christian Science Wednesday Night healing sessions. Such healings could well be produced by the patient's mental state, faith, or belief. The group setting and participants at such healing sessions can add much to the power of suggestion.

Although it is still too early to describe with certainty the physiological mechanism by which behavior, belief, and faith promote healing, there is now clear and irrefutable evidence that the central nervous system and the immune system are involved. These two systems of the body communicate regularly with each other. The cells of the immune system have well-developed receptors for neuropeptides — those important chemicals of the brain that are active in the transmission of brain messages.

One fundamental characteristic of the cells of both the nervous and immune systems is their capacity for memory. In sensitized lymphocytes of the immune system is the memory that permits the antigen/antibody reaction, which is the basis of the allergic reaction. Memory function is essential to life and the body's antigen/antibody response that is essential to healing. Stress management interventions such as relaxation, anxiety reduction and social support have all been found to improve immune functions. Solid evidence exists from several laboratories that an increase in serum concentration of essential brain chemicals, especially the endogenous opioids, have direct effects on immunity.

The right half of the brain is the seat of emotional thinking. It is here that religious music would have a great influence. Beliefs here are not easily influenced by logic. Here then would be the ideal candidate for the anatomical location of religious thought. In the right hemisphere, ideas are translated into images for action upon the autonomic nervous system. The autonomic system is that part of the nervous system that responds to emotion, keeps the body in homeostatic balance, and which, with disruption, can be responsible for disease.

Imagery has always played a key role in the practice of medicine and has in itself therapeutic significance (24). Clinically, imagery has been used to stimulate the body's healing by its action in strengthening the immune system. This has been demonstrated by surgeon Bernie Siegal (25), the Simontons (26), and others who use imagery as a tool in the battle against cancer. Social support is one mainstay of religious belonging. The importance of congregations as primary social groups, giving identity and improvement in self-image, undoubtedly plays an important role in promoting health, healing, improved body image, and a sense of well-being.

On the physical side, certain brain peptides are important. They play an essential role in controlling pain, promoting relaxation, and controlling emotions. These are the enkephalins and endorphins, which also play a role in imagery. The placebo effect is a dramatic example of imagination in action, a mechanism mediated by endorphins. This relationship of endorphins to the immune system and of Beta-endorphin to the imagination and imagery suggests the powerful link that occurs between faith and body physiology. Lasagna and co-workers (27) found a markedly higher percentage of placebo-positive persons among regular church-goers than among non-churchgoers. In view of the foregoing discussion, do we now have evidence of a biological mechanism by which a strong faith in God could be translated into a healing of the body?

## REFERENCES

1. Rose, L. (1968). *Faith healing.* New York: Penguin Books.
2. Rose, L. (1954). Some aspects of paranormal healing. *Brit Med J, 4900,* 1329-1332.
3. Dossey, L. (1993). *Healing words. The power of prayer and the practice of medicine.* New York: Harper.
4. Byrd, R. (1988). Positive therapeutic effects of intercessory prayer

in a coronary care unit population. *Southern Med J, 81/7*, 826-829.
5. Dakin, E. (1929). *Mrs. Eddy*. New York: Blue Ribbon Books.
6. Enroth, R. (1992). *Churches that abuse*. Grand Rapids, MI: Zondervan.
7. Chiribin, J. (1992). Healing and spirituality. *Pastoral Psychol, 40* (4), 235-244.
8. Kua, E.; Che, P.; & Ko, S. Spirit possession and healing among Chinese psychiatric patients. *Acta Psychiatr Scand 88*, 447-450.
9. Henry, W.; Sims, H.; & Spray, S. (1971). *The fifth profession*. San Francisco, CA: Jessey-Base.
10. Larson, D. (1985). Religious involvement. In G. Rekers (Ed.), *Family building*. Ventura, CA: Regal.
11. Larson, D., & Larson, S. (1991). Religious commitment and health: Valuing the relationship. *Second Opinion: Health, Faith and Ethics, 17* (1), 26-40.
12. Witmer, J., & Zimmerman, M. (1991). Intercessory prayer as medical treatment? An inquiry. *Skeptical Inquirer, 15*, 177-180.
13. *Alcoholics Anonymous*. (1947). Cornwall, NY: Cornwall Press.
14. Larson, D., & Wilson, W. (1980). Religious life of alcoholics. *Southern Med J, 73* (6),723-727.
15. Gartner, J.; Larson, D.; & Allen, G. (1991). Religious commitment and mental health. A review of the empirical literature. *J Psychol and Theol, 19*(1), 6-25.
16. Comstock, G., & Partridge, K. (1972). Church attendance and health. *J Chron Dis, 25*, 665-672.
17. Argyle, M., & Beit-Hallahami, B. (1975). *The social psychology of religion*. London: Routledge & Kegan Paul.
18. Tavris, C., & Sadd, S. (1977). *The Redbook report on female sexuality*. New York: Delacorte Press.
19. Levin, J., & Vanderpool, H. (1989). Is religion therapeutically significant for hypertension? *Soc Sci Med, 29* (1), 69-78.
20. Levin, J., & Schiller, P. (1987). Is there a religious factor in faith? *J Rel and Health, 24*(7), 589-600.
21. Spiegel, D. (1991). A psychosocial intervention and survival time of patients with metastatic breast cancer. Symington Foundation Sym-

posium. New directions in cancer care (1990, Summer) *Advances, 3*, 10-19.
22. Beecher, H. (1955). The powerful placebo. *JAMA , 159*, 1602-1604.
23. Neame, A. (1967). *The happening at Lourdes*. New York: Simon & Schuster.
24. Achterberg, J. (1985). *Imagery in healing*. Boston: New Science Library.
25. Siegel, B. (1990). *Peace, love and healing. Bodymind communication and the path to self-healing. An exploration*. New York: Harper.
26. Simonton, O. C., et al. (1978). *Getting well again*. Los Angeles, CA: Tarche.
27. Lasagna, L., et al. (1954). A study of the placebo response. *Amer J Med, 16*, 77-79.

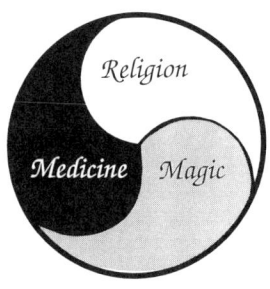

# V

# THE MANY FACES OF RELAXATION

RELAXATION is an integral factor in most holistic treatment methods. In Ayurvedic medicine, it is achieved by yogic postures and meditation; in Chinese medicine, it is the slow relaxing movements of external *Qi Gong*, *Tai ch'i* and martial arts that bring balance to the "forces of *Yin* and *Yang*." Hypnosis combines relaxation with concentration to create the "trance." Biofeedback is itself a form of relaxation. The naturopath, chiropractor, and osteopath frequently recommend various types of relaxing treatments to achieve what the allopathic physician does with a prescription for Valium.

Claude Bernard (1813-78) (1) introduced the term "homeostasis," referring to those forces that bring about a stable internal psychological and physiological state within the body — a state of wellness. Walter Cannon's book, *Bodily Changes in Pain, Hunger, Fear and Rage* (1929) (2), describes the interaction of the two opposing parts of the autonomic nervous system, the sympathetic and parasympathetic divisions. It is the sympathetic that, in response to stress, causes the blood pressure to rise, the heart to race, breathing to become rapid, and the pupils to dilate. The parasympathetic has the opposite response, producing relaxation.

Cannon termed the sympathetic reaction the "fight or flight" response to external stressors. This was vital to the survival of our ancestors, who needed the body to become energized in order to escape from or successfully conquer their enemies. As humankind became more "civilized," the enemy moved "within." It then was worry, anguish, and anxiety about untoward events that produced inner stress. The bodily adjustments for "fight or flight" were no longer appropriate for dealing with an internalized stress created by environmental pressures. Yet they persist. As Selye (3) and others pointed out and is now general knowledge, prolonged stress leads to illness. Relaxation is the opposite of stress; hence, it is a prophylactic method for preventing and, in some cases, healing the various stress-produced diseases.

Edmond Jacobsen, a Chicago physiologist (4), reported that the thought of a muscle movement produced action in the nerves leading to that muscle. He introduced a method known as **progressive relaxation.** In this, the muscles are first tensed maximally and then relaxed in order to teach the body the sensations of tension preceding the process of relaxation. Jacobsen's method of progressive relaxation was quickly adopted by psychiatry as a means of treating anxiety and neurotic states before psychoactive drugs were available. In his book, *You Must Relax* (1934) (5), Jacobsen recommended his method not only for nervous disorders, but for insomnia, digestive complaints, and high blood pressure as well.

Johannes Schultz, a German psychiatrist interested in hypnosis, developed the system of **autogenic training** (6) in the 1930's. In this method, without the use of hypnosis but through a series of exercises, the patient reaches a deep state of relaxation. There are six states of the exercise: heaviness, warmth, regulation of the heartbeat, regulation of respiration, abdominal warmth, and finally, head cooling. This is followed by a series of meditative exercises. Schultz recommended the clinical application of his autogenic training relaxation methods for numerous ailments, including respiratory, gastrointestinal, cardiovascular, endocrine, urogenital, sexual, dermatological, insomnia, nervous diseases including convulsions, and all types of psychiatric disturbances.

In 1975, Herbert Benson, a cardiologist, coined the term "**relaxation response**," described in a book with the same title (7). Benson had become interested in the yogic use of the repetition of a secret word or *mantra* accompanied by rhythmic breathing to produce a state of relaxation. He was fascinated by reports of Zen masters who could lower their blood pressure and slow their heart rate through meditation. He later found that any neutral word or meaningless syllable monotonously repeated was effective. Even more effective was the use of a prayer or inspirational phrase that had some spiritual significance for the patient. The essential ingredients of Benson's method are: *1)* sit comfortably, relaxed and with eyes closed; *2)* breathe deeply into the abdominal area; *3)* silently repeat one word as you exhale or focus on breathing; *4)* if any intrusive thoughts occur, refocus on the breathing; and *5)* repeat once or twice daily for 10-20 minutes.

Some elaborate systems of relaxation use **isolation tanks**, either dry or filled with water. In the latter, the person enjoys the sensation of floating while lying in six or eight inches of water. These tanks are, in essence, small soundproof rooms, devoid of changes in light and darkness. The temperature is kept neutral. In the tanks, the water is at skin temperature. Unlike the previously described methods, isolation techniques require no effort on the part of the individual, but they are more costly than the simpler methods. Also used are methods that emphasize **visual imagery**, usually of past scenes, places where the patient has experienced feelings of comfort and relaxation.

Techniques such as *reiki*, therapeutic touch, massage, hypnosis, biofeedback, and others contain within them a state of quiet relaxation for the person being treated. From the research point of view, it is thus often difficult to determine just how much many of such healing techniques rely on relaxation in their effort to induce homeostasis. Relaxed states can enhance healing by counteracting anxiety with its accompanying widespread tension that interferes with all body functions (8).

Add relaxation to the placebo effect and there is a combined action that can enhance immune functions. Relaxation then may well be the essential component that underlies many of the techniques of alternative medicine.

## Biofeedback

*Feedback* occurs when a system controls and corrects itself by reviewing results of past performance. It has long aided the tennis coach and the piano teacher. The woman straightening her posture in front of a mirror is using feedback; so is the jogger checking his pulse as he runs. Its systematic and scientific application to disordered biological systems is a reasonable and useful technique.

*Biofeedback* refers to the human capacity to augment proprioceptive or interoceptive sensory information mechanically. It employs electronic sensors that give visual or auditory signals to inform the subject of changes in biological processes of which the individual is normally unaware, i.e., heart rate, muscle tension, etc. The underlying hypothesis is that if someone can be made aware of bodily processes of which s/he is not usually conscious, s/he can then learn to control these functions. With biofeedback techniques, persons learn to influence bodily responses ordinarily not under voluntary control or to regulate the processes which are ordinarily well-regulated but are malfunctioning due to disease or trauma.

The biofeedback technique augments proprioception and interoception in three ways:
- By changing the perception to a more familiar or more usable form, such as a visual display in place of a dull visceral sensation.
- By making the signal more intense such as a clear sound of varying pitch in place of a weak biological signal.
- By pairing the sensations with a continuously changing numerical "score."

It is to be recognized that biofeedback is not itself a complete treatment but rather a technique used in an overall therapeutic approach that may well involve psychotherapy, medication, and relaxation training. Biofeedback is conducted in a quiet room free from outside distractions. With electronic monitors attached, the patient relaxes, usually in a comfortable chair. S/he focuses on his body sensations, but in a neutral, passive way, focusing on a mental representation of the "target sensation" that s/he hopes to achieve. Treatments are given once or twice a week with instructions to practice at home. Sessions are of 20-45 minutes duration. The number of sessions required depends on the patient and the problem being treated.

Historically, attempts to intensify self-awareness were highly developed in the Orient, using meditation techniques often with religious connotations. This approach to mind/body medicine, with prolonged periods of practice, often resulted in impressive degrees of self-control, as demonstrated by Buddhists and the Yogis of India.

In the West, forerunners of biofeedback included not only the meditations and prayers of the early Judeo-Christian religion, but also the techniques of hypnosis, progressive relaxation, autogenic training, and auto-analysis. Technical advances in the recording of physiological responses — including the EKG, EEG, polygraph, and more recently, the computer — made possible modern biofeedback.

EEG biofeedback techniques were pioneered by Dr. Joseph Kamiya of San Francisco (9). Since then, the use of biofeedback has spread widely. There is now a professional society, The Association for Applied Psychophysiology and Biofeedback, with affiliated organizations in many of the states and similar societies in Canada, Australia, and elsewhere. Elmer and Alyce Green of Topeka, Kansas, (10) pioneered a biofeedback hand-warming technique for the treatment of migraine headaches. They also travelled to India, monitoring Yogis who claimed that through meditation they could regulate their nervous systems and metabolic rates. In the last three decades, biofeedback has developed a degree of scientific respectability, with research published in refereed journals. Despite this, however, and due especially to claims regarding the relationship of biofeedback to states of altered consciousness, some scientific controversy still remains.

The most commonly used types of biofeedback are as follows:

***Thermal Biofeedback.*** This involves monitoring skin temperature in order to increase (warm) or decrease (cool) blood flow in the extremities. A temperature-measuring device on the finger feeds information back to the patient, who through imagery and relaxation gradually learns to control body temperature. This type of biofeedback is used in the treatment of Raynaud's disease, in which blood vessels in the fingers and toes constrict painfully in cold weather. It has been applied successfully to patients with migraine headaches when increases and decreases in cerebral blood flow may be a causative factor. Such use presumes a generalization of the effect from peripheral blood vessels to intracranial blood vessels. This effect has not been proven, suggesting that the demonstrated success in treating headache may be due in part to the training in relaxation that occurs during the biofeedback procedures.

While most persons cannot unaided detect changes of 5.0 degrees Fahrenheit, with biofeedback training which monitors changes of as little as 0.01 degree, patients can learn to judge hand temperature with accuracy and to raise hand temperature to within 5 degrees of core body temperature.

***Electromyographic Biofeedback.*** Here the monitor is an electromyograph which measures the electrical activity in muscles, reflecting the degree of tension in the muscle that is being studied. This method is used in pain clinics to address maladaptive muscular habits often developed by patients in response to continuing symptoms of pain (i.e.. bracing, guarding). Tense muscles contract and can sometimes cause pressure upon nerves, thus intensifying the pain. This suggests that there can be benefit from the muscular relaxation that is mediated by EMG biofeedback. Most often, the site of EMG monitoring is directly related to the individual's muscular problem or specific area of pain.

Biofeedback has been successful for the treatment of tension and migraine headaches, for bruxism, torticollis and low back pain. It has been used in neuromuscular rehabilitation to re-establish disrupted and functionally atrophied sensory-motor feedback systems in patients, following both upper and lower motor neuron injury.

*Electrodermal Biofeedback.* The electrodermal biofeedback device, abbreviated as EDR or GSR, is an important part of polygraph testing. It measures changes in skin conductance associated with sweating. The polygraph has been widely used in investigative work, where it is felt that the secrets of persons hiding damaging evidence behind a calm facade may be exposed by the telltale reaction of the autonomic nervous system. Such measurements, however, are subject to false interpretations and hence their evidential use has been rejected by many courts.

Electrodermal biofeedback has also been used in the treatment of anxiety, panic states, phobias, excessive sweating, and stuttering on the premise that reducing autonomic arousal can decrease the physical discomfort that may serve to precipitate or exacerbate feelings of anxiety.

*Other Somatic Biofeedback.* Devices to monitor blood pressure and heartbeat have been used to treat cardiac patients with hypertension and cardiac dysrhythmias. Patients can significantly reduce premature ventricular contractions and maintain the benefit for years. Biofeedback techniques have been used to assist patients with asthma, bowel dysfunction, and acidity of the stomach.

Physiological relaxation responses associated with autonomic calming can also be learned through imagery and other relaxation techniques (11). Biofeedback monitoring can document the effect of other such relaxation techniques. In this manner, it can be used by athletes to moderate pre-game apprehension. According to Dr. Barbara Brown, "Any body function that can be measured quite precisely and fairly continuously can be trained to come under voluntary control." (12)

***Electroencephalographic Biofeedback.*** EEG biofeedback utilizes the electroencephalograph to monitor brain wave activity while the patient sits quietly with eyes closed with electrodes affixed to the scalp. Alpha waves (8-13 cycles per second activity) accompany relaxation. This method was initially used for the treatment of anxiety.

In the late 1960's, claims were made that alpha waves were indicators of meditation or psychic states. This spawned a multi-million dollar business in the sale of portable alpha-feedback machines for home use. The promotion of such equipment overlooks the fact that proper recording of the EEG requires costly equipment with artifact resistant electrodes meticulously applied and electronic shielding to eliminate pervasive environmental electromagnetic noise. Home recording often becomes invalid through contamination of the record by the spurious recording of higher amplitude heart, skin, muscle, and eye movement potentials. Hence, such units are impractical.

Alpha waves are related to visual activity of the occipital cortex. They are "blocked" by opening the eyes and disappear with attention or mental effort. Statements linking alpha waves to mental states arose from observations in Japan and India, reporting that experienced Zen and Yoga meditators showed much alpha in their EEG's, even with their eyes open. The frequent mistake of attributing cause to events that are simply associational was made here. There was a failure to account for the fact that such highly trained individuals during the state of meditation were not processing visual information and had developed the ability to ignore stimuli that usually block alpha.

The enthusiastic reception accorded to the belief that alpha was related to transpersonal events was part of a worldwide interest in "New Age" phenomena. In reality, there has been little scientific evidence to warrant such over-enthusiasm. In many of the published reports, little attention was given to errors that could occur with baseline (before training) measurements. Novelty, excitement, and anxiety on a first exposure to the laboratory all tend to lower the amount of alpha in the EEG. With the aid of eyes-open feedback training of focusing and attentional attitudes, the subject can gradually overcome such alpha blocking. Johnson (13) concluded that there has never been a conclusive demonstration of learned enhancement of alpha in excess of a true eyes-closed baseline.

While abundant alpha is seen at times of relaxation, this does not necessarily imply that alpha can produce relaxation. Beyerstein (14) and others have reported that persons with high levels of anxiety may demonstrate high levels of alpha.

The wide acceptance of alpha-biofeedback training is indicative of an unmet need for adequate therapies to control such complaints as insomnia, anxiety, tension headaches, and similar afflictions. Many reports of therapeutic benefit suffer from the neglect of placebo controls. A controlled study by Melzack and Wall (15) concluded that for the amelioration of pain, such techniques as relaxation and coping-skills training are equivalent to biofeedback.

Attention has recently turned to theta wave biofeedback as the royal road to transpersonal experiences. That segment of the electroencephalographic spectrum in the range of 4-7 cycles per second is designated as theta activity. Such waves are common in reverie as one becomes drowsy, and they precede the appearance of the slow delta wave ($\frac{1}{2}$ - 3 cycles) activity of sleep. For this reason, biofeedback training to produce these slower patterns has been used in the treatment of insomnia.

Most recently, biofeedback training to produce alpha-theta brain rhythms has been proposed by Peniston and Kulkosky (16) as an adjunct in the treatment of alcoholism. Some claim that it decreases the amount of peripheral B-endorphin that increases with anxiety and is a common feature in chronic alcoholics. In reviewing research on theta activity, Johnson (13) concludes that theta in the human EEG is "an artifact of general lowering of arousal level."

Recent attention has turned to the use of EEG or neurofeedback in the treatment of attention deficit hyperactivity disorder. Although good results are reported with this intervention, the treatment is lengthy, requiring as many as 40 visits.

In current biofeedback treatment, the modalities used are individualized and relevant for each patient. The sites for monitoring are specific for the presenting symptoms. A great deal of attention is placed on generalization of skills to the home environment. Behavior therapy is usually incorporated to assist the patient in developing self-regulation strategies (17). A unique advantage of biofeedback over general relaxation is its ability to focus on the specific system and area of dysfunction.

## Hypnosis

Hypnosis is an ancient method of healing with a colorful but somewhat checkered history (18). Early civilizations in Egypt and Greece had sleep temples, while India and the Far East had Holy Men who induced trances and demonstrated unusual control over their sensory and motor processes. Priests in the temple of Aesculapius, 400 C.E., induced hypnotic sleep. The Judeo-Christian Bible tells of Adam's "hypnotic anesthesia" for the birth of Eve.

The modern era of hypnosis began with **Franz Anton Mesmer** (1734-1815), a German mystic who as a medical student wrote his thesis, *De Planatarium Influx,* about a strange magnetic fluid, the poor distribution of which produced disease. He later came to believe that a kind of "animal magnetism" emanated from his hands and could produce a "crisis" followed by healing. His strange practices and his indiscretion with a young female patient led to his ouster from Vienna. He moved to Paris, where he established a healing salon. In 1784, Louis XVI appointed a committee which included Benjamin Franklin to investigate Mesmer. They returned a report stating that his cures resulted not from any mysterious body energy or magnetism, but rather from suggestion.

**Marquis de Puysegur** (1751-1825), a disciple of Mesmer, reported that the "crises" were unnecessary, and he induced a sleep-like trance and somnambulism by passes of his hand.

**Abbe Faria** (1756-1819), a wandering Portuguese monk, had learned in India how to produce a somnambulistic trance by simply gazing into a subjects' eyes and shouting loudly, "Sleep!" **Alexander Bertrand** (1795-1831) claimed that hypnosis was a psychological phenomenon due to suggestion. **John Elliotson** (1791-1868), professor of medicine at London University, used hypnosis in the treatment of medical and nervous disorders and as an anesthetic. **James Esdaile** (1808-1895), a Scottish surgeon, read of Elliotson's work and, as head of a special hospital in Calcutta, India, performed several thousand operations under hypnosis.

**James Braid** (1795-1860), a physician in Manchester, England, conducted studies on catalepsy and amnesia. He used this method to treat rheumatism, paralysis, and neuralgia, and renamed the process "hypnosis," from the Greek *hypnos*, meaning sleep. **A. A. Liebeault** (1823-1904), a country physician in Nancy, France, became acquainted with

Braid's book *Neurypnology or the Rationale of Nervous Sleep, Considered in Relation with Animal Magnetism* and added verbal suggestions to the method of eye fixation. He formed a clinic and treated hundreds of patients by this method. **Hippolyte Bernheim** (1837-1919), a professor of medicine at Strasbourg, was originally skeptical of Liebeault's work, but later joined him to form the Nancy School, which stressed the psychological nature of these treatments.

**Jean Martin Charcot** (1825-1893), professor of neurology at the Salpetriere Hospital in Paris, opposed the psychological theories of the Nancy school and proposed that hypnosis was physically caused and was a pathological manifestation of hysteria. He described hypnosis as having three stages: lethargic, cataleptic, and somnambulistic. His prestige was great and he influenced many thinkers. **Joseph Breuer** (1841-1925), a Viennese physician, proposed that the symptoms of hysteria were the outgrowth of forgotten past events. He utilized hypnosis to enhance the recall of such forgotten memories. **Sigmund Freud** (1856-1939), also of Vienna, studied with Charcot and at the Nancy school. He attempted to use hypnosis for the recall of forgotten memories but was unsuccessful and abandoned hypnosis in favor of the free-association techniques of psychoanalysis.

**Pierre Janet** (1859-1947), professor of psychology at the College of France, demonstrated that suggestive therapy rightly belonged with other treatment methods in psychiatry. **Boris Sidis** (1854-1929) supported belief in the therapeutic efficacy of a light state of hypnosis. **Emile Coue** (1857-1926), a young druggist who studied under Liebeault, used waking suggestions as a means of autosuggestion. He instructed his patients to use a knotted string after the fashion of a rosary and to repeat, "Every day, in every way, I feel better and better." **Morton Prince** (1854-1929), founder of the Harvard Psychological Clinic, reported on the use of hypnosis for the study of multiple personality.

The modern era of experimental investigations of hypnosis owes much to the publications of **Clark Hull** (1933), professor of psychology at Yale. However, just as gas inhalation anesthesia appeared on the medical scene in 1846 at a time inimical to the use of hypnosis, so the rise in popularity of psychoanalysis delayed the integration of hypnosis into psychiatric treatment for another half century. But, as predicted by Janet, "If my book be ignored today, it will be read tomorrow, when there will have been a new turn of fashion's wheel, bringing back treatment by hypnotic suggestion just as it will bring back our Grandmothers' hats."

In World War I, **J.A. Hadfield** used "hypnoanalysis" in the treatment of shell-shocked soldiers. **Lewis Wolberg** emphasized the integration of hypnosis and dynamic psychiatry in his two-volume work published in 1948. Experiences of World War II showed the need for more efficient methods of treating psychiatric casualties, and a number of publications appeared on the therapeutic applications of hypnosis in the military setting by **Horsley, Gringer** and **Spiegel, Brenman** and **Gill, Erickson** and others.

In 1948, the British Society of Medical Hypnosis was formed, followed by the publication of the *British Journal of Medical Hypnosis*. The Society for Clinical and Experimental Hypnosis was founded in the United States in 1949, followed in 1953 by the publication of the *Journal of Clinical and Experimental Hypnosis*. In 1957, the American Society of Clinical Hypnosis was formed with its journal the *American Journal of Clinical Hypnosis*. In 1958, the Council on Mental Health of the American Medical Association gave official status to hypnotism as a therapeutic adjunct under responsible medical and dental direction.

**The Nature of Hypnosis**

Hypnosis may be defined as the uncritical acceptance of a suggestion. Suggestions may come from different sources and may be verbal or non-verbal, deliberate or inadvertent. Youth, reasonably high intelligence, and the personality trait of amiability seem to be associated with hypnotizability, a trait which falls on the usual bell-shaped curve of biological characteristics. Hypnotizable persons seem better able than others to focus their attention on the defined subject matter and disregard distracting stimuli. Hypnosis has been simply defined as a state of relaxation and concentration, in which a very special relationship exists between the hypnotist and the hypnotized subject, who is able to do, think, feel, believe, and remember whatever the hypnotist suggests.

A considerable difference of opinion exists as to whether there is a physiologically definable "trance state." Descriptions of such a state have varied from the "crises" of Mesmer, the sleep and somnambulism of Puysegar, the anesthesia of Elliotson, the three stages of Charcot, and the waking hypnosis of the Nancy school. Hypnosis appears to include all of the above, varying only with the intent of the hypnotist, the beliefs of the subject and the nature of the occasion, for in the end all hypnosis is self-induced in the manner of the belief of the hypnotized. Recently, a number of hypnotists (19, 20, 21) have supported the belief that hypnosis is a form of "role-taking" behavior, determined at least in part by social-psychological pressures. The success of the hypnotic procedure is thus dependent upon the subjects' expectancies, their aptitude for role taking, and their perception of the role expected of a hypnotized person. The subject behaves as he/she thinks a hypnotized person should act, and thus shapes the experience.

The debate still continues over whether hypnotic phenomena are best explained by a social/psychological interpretation in which the behavior seen is a voluntary response, or whether it is a special process in which so-called "good hypnotic subjects" have lost their control over behavior induced by suggestion.

In the experimental laboratory, amnesics do in fact retain control over retrieval processes and accommodate their lack of control to the social demands of the experimental situation. Likewise with experimental pain, subjects rendered analgesic by hypnosis report a subjective reduction of pain while their body's subconscious physiological reaction is that characteristically seen accompanying a noxious stimulus. Hilgard has termed this phenomenon the "hidden observer." (22)

We now know that information can be independently processed in different parts of the brain and not necessarily communicated to other parts of the brain. Contemporary dissociation theories now support biological explanations for Post-Traumatic Stress Disorders and for Multiple Personality Disorder. Socially influenced behavior can have a neural component. The right hemisphere may have a preferential role in the capacity for trance expression (23).

Our early EEG research (24) showed that high hypnotizables had an increase in fast (Beta) activity. Later research by Sabourin et al. (25) showed that highly susceptible subjects had more beta activity in the left than in the right hemispheres, while low susceptible subjects showed only weak asymmetry. Crawford (26) quotes Hilgard, reporting that when a person experiences complete anesthesia for pain following hypnotic suggestions, there is still ongoing, unrecognized, physiological reactivity. Blood pressure, galvanic skin conductance, and the earlier sensory components of somatosensory-evoked potentials continue to indicate physiological reactivity, yet distress and sensory pain are nonexistent. The highs act somewhat like lobotomized patients, who often report sensory pain but without the presence of the distress component. This suggests that hypnotic analgesia is a function of the far fronto-limbic attentional system, "deciding" or "directing" the thalamic cortical system to acknowledge and then disattend the pain messages. Using cerebral blood flow techniques, Crawford et al. (26) showed dramatic differences between low and high hypnotizables. The anterior temporal region, particularly on the right side, and the far frontal cortex showed substantially greater cerebral metabolic activity in the highly hypnotizable, while they successfully turned off all pain perception. Recently, Crawford (27) has shown with topographical mapping of the cortex in response to evoked potentials, a demonstration that hypnotic analgesia reduces the sensory responsiveness of the posterior pain system and shows a dramatic diminution of activity in the far frontal region. In summary, her research suggests that the far frontal cortex is differentially activated during hypnotic analgesia. The "executive controller" acts as a gate against the ascent of thalamic activity (processing pain) to the cortex so that it cannot be interpreted at a cognitive level. During hypnotic analgesia, the far frontal cortex "determines" that the incoming painful events are irrelevant and inhibits somatosensory information coming from the thalamic region.

In real-life clinical situations, one sees under hypnosis events not seen in the experimental laboratory. For example, in the case of severe pain during the debridement of extensive burns in children (28), hypnosis can modulate pain far beyond the level seen in the laboratory where someone is to be obeyed or impressed. Spiegel et al. (29) have demonstrated the suppression of cortical-evoked responses in patients with hypnotically induced visual hallucinations.

In developed countries, the soil is unripe among highly educated persons for spontaneously arising "visions" and other paranormal imagery once commonly reported in more primitive societies. In those days, the hypnotic state was more colorful. Today, the skepticism that prompted Benjamin Franklin to attribute Mesmer's claims to suggestion is more prevalent. The issue, then, is not just one of state versus trait, but rather which capabilities for hypnotic responsiveness are biologically innate and which are more environmentally sensitive and determined by the social climate.

**Induction Techniques**

The general principles of induction techniques include a variety of methods for restricting the perceptual field in persons who desire to receive suggestions. In our book (18), we have emphasized that a good hypnotic subject exhibits the trait of "amiability," thus entering the desired state by whatever means the hypnotist suggests. One of the keys to successful hypnotic induction, however, is matching the technique to the personality of the patient, to the setting, and to the purpose of the hypnosis. Techniques vary with different hypnotists, from those who emphasize the physical such as arm-raising, or the eye-roll maneuver (30) to those who use indirect, verbal, and non-verbal techniques that lead the patient into a hypnotic state through conversational methods which subtly imply the type of behavioral goals desired (31).

The progressive relaxation techniques of Jacobsen (32) can serve as a form of hypnotic induction. This method is more elaborately demonstrated through the Autogenic Training of Johannes Schultz (33), in which the subject is taken through a program of mental exercises.

The old ideas that persons might not awaken from the "trance," or that they can be controlled by the hypnotist or hypnotized to do things against their will are still suggested by stage hypnotists and movies but are definitely untrue.

**Uses of Hypnosis**

Hypnosis is one of the best documented psychological techniques for controlling acute and chronic pain in adults and children (34, 28). It is also beneficial in reducing insomnia associated with chronic pain (35), tinnitus (36), and certain sleep disorders (37). In controlled clinical trial studies, hypnosis intervention for pain has been found to be equal to or more effective than biofeedback, autogenic training, and cognitive behavioral training (38). Yet, hypnosis for pain management is underemployed compared to other modalities, probably due to a combination of factors, including misconceptions about hypnosis by both health professionals and the general public, limited training opportunities for physicians, and lack of understanding of the neuropsychophysiological foundations of hypnosis and hypnotic analgesia. Kroger (39) and others have promoted the use of hypnosis for the relief of pain and assistance in the process of childbirth.

Hypnosis has been useful in reducing the severe nausea and side effects of chemotherapy for cancer (40). Speigel and his associates (41) found that women with breast cancer who had participated in support groups that included self-hypnosis had a significantly longer life expectancy. Hypnosis has been successfully used for both recurrent tension and migraine-type headaches (28). It has been used with burn patients undergoing painful debridement (42). It is a successful treatment technique for musculoskeletal disorders, including low back pain and fibromyalgia (35).

Hypnosis has long been used for the cure of warts, with direct suggestion proving successful in 27-55% of reported cases. Here, however, and in correcting such unwanted occurrences as nosebleeds, it appears that indirect suggestions are better. For example, to quell the flow of blood, one might be told to imagine a cake of ice on the nose rather than be given the direction for the nose to "stop bleeding." Or, when warts are made to disappear, the suggestion could be to imagine a temperature change or something that would cause an alteration in the blood flow to the skin around the warts. With children, rubbing the wart with a "magic penny" is an often recommended technique.

Demonstrations of hypnotically induced "board-like" rigidity are used by stage hypnotists when persons are suspended between the backs of two chairs while resting only on their neck and ankles. This appears startling, but has nothing to do with a supposed hypnotically induced state of super strength. Under the proper circumstances, any slightly built person can do this trick. Feats of supernormal ability have been reported by many persons in emergency situations where seemingly superhuman efforts are required to save a life.

In the field of psychiatry, hypnosis has been used to recall forgotten memories. It has been useful in the treatment of dissociation in multiple personality and in post-traumatic stress disorders. Extravagant statements about bringing back memories of a previous existence and the so-called regression of an adult to an "actual state" of childhood result from vivid imagination and an adeptness at role-playing by the hypnotized person. In such cases, changes in the EEG under hypnosis simply reflect the depth of relaxation or drowsiness.

As the hypnotic state is often characterized by a concentration of attention accompanied by profound relaxation, it can be a useful technique for patients who are under stress or have anxiety disorders or psychosomatic illnesses aggravated by stress.

It is important to remember that hypnosis is not itself a treatment but only a technique that can enhance treatment procedures used in various specialties of medicine or dentistry. The concept of "hypnotist" is to be avoided, as hypnosis is not a "cure-all" but a technique that can be beneficially applied by persons working within their own specialty who elect to use hypnosis where it is useful and appropriate.

## REFERENCES

1. Bernard, C. (1880). *Lecons de physologie experimental appliques a la medicine au College de France.* Paris, France: J. E. Bailliere et fils.
2. Cannon, W. (1932).*Wisdom of the body.* New York: W.W.Norton.
3. Selye, H. (1956). *The Stress of life.* New York: McGraw Hill.
4. Jacobsen, E. (1938). *Progressive relaxation.* Chicago: University of Chicago Press.
5. Jacobsen, E. (1934). *You must relax.* New York: McGraw Hill.
6. Schultz, J. & Luthe, W. (1959). *Autogenic training:A psychophysiologic approach in psychotherapy.* New York: Grune & Stratton.
7. Benson, H. (1975). *The relaxation response.* New York: Avon Books.
8. National Institutes of Health Technology Assessment Conference Statement. (October 16-18, 1995). *Integration of behavioral and relaxation approaches into the treatment of chronic pain and insomnia.* Kensington, MD: NIH Consensus Program Information Service.
9. Kamiya, J. (1969). Operant control of the EEG alpha rhythm and some of its reported effects on consciousness. In C. Tart (Ed.), *Altered States of Consciousness.* New York: Anchor Books.

10. Green, E., & Green, A. (1986). Biofeedback and states of consciousness. In B. Wolman & M. Ullman (Eds.), *Handbook of states of consciouness*. New York: Van Nostrand Reinhold.
11. Thomas, R., et al. (1993). The effects of biofeedback on carpal tunnel syndrome. *Ergonomics, 36,* 353-361.
12. Brown, B. (1974). *New mind, new body*. New York: Harper and Row.
13. Johnson, L. (1977). Learned control of brain activity. In J. Beatty & H. Legewie (Eds.), *Biofeedback and behavior*. New York: Plenum Press.
14. Beyerstein, B. (1985). The myth of alpha consciousness. *Skeptical Inquirer, 10,* 42-59.
15. Melzack, R., & Wall, P. (1982). *The challenge of pain*. Harmondsworth: Penguin.
16. Peniston, E., & Kulkosky, P. (1989). Alpha-theta brainwave training and b-endorphin levels in alcoholics. *Alcoholism – Clinical and Experimental Research, 13,* 271-279.
17. Schwartz, M. (1987). *Biofeedback: A practitioner's handbook*. New York: Guilford Press.
18. Ulett, G., & Peterson, D. (1965). *Applied hypnosis and positive suggestion*. St. Louis: C.V. Mosby.
19. Barber, T.X. (1964). Hypnotizability, suggestibility and personality: Part V: A critical reveiw of research findings. *Psychol Rep, 14,* 229-320. Monograph supp. 3-V14.
20. Sarbin, T. (1950). Contributions to role-taking theory in hypnotic behavior. *Psychol Rev, 57,* 255-270.
21. Orne, M. (1959). The nature of hypnosis: Artifact and essence. *J Abnorm Soc Psychol, 58,* 277-299.
22. Hilgard, E. (1986). *Divided consciousness: Multiple controls in human thought and action*. New York: Wiley.
23. Gur, R., & Gur, R. (1974). Handedness, sex and eyedness as moderating variables in the relation between hypnotic susceptibility and functional brain asymmetry. *J Abnorm Psychol, 83,* 635-643.
24. Ulett, G.; Akpinar, S.; & Itil, T. (1972). Hypnosis: physiological, pharmacological reality. *Amer J Psychiat, 128,* 33-339.

25. Sabourin, M., et al. (1990). EEG correlates of hypnotic susceptibility and hypnotic trance: Spectral analysis and coherence. *Int J Psychophysiol, 120,* 125-142.
26. Crawford, H.; Brown, A.; & Moon, C. (1993). Sustained attentional and disattentional abilities. Differences between low and high hypnotizables. *J Abnorm Psychol, 102* (4), 534-543.
27. Crawford, H.; & Gruzelier, J. (1992). A midstream view of the neuropsychophysiology of hypnosis: Recent research and future direction. In Fromm & Nash (Eds.), *Contemporary hypnosis research.* New York: Guilford Press.
28. Hilgard, E., & Hilgard, J. (1994). *Hypnosis in the relief of pain* (rev. ed.). New York: Brunner/Mazel.
29. Spiegel, D.; Bierre, P.; & Rootenberg, J. (1989). Hypnotic alteration of somatosensory perception: Accompanying changes in evoked potentials. *Amer J Psychiat, 146,* 749-754.
30. Spiegel, H., & Spiegel, D. (1978). *Trance and treatment.* New York: Basic Books.
31. Haley, J. (1967). *Advanced techniques of hypnosis and therapy: Selected papers of Milton H. Erickson, M.D.* New York: Grune & Stratton.
32. Jacobsen, E. (1938). *Progressive relaxation.* Chicago: University Chicago Press.
33. Schulz, J., & Luthe, W. (1959). *Autogenic training: A psychophysiologic approach to psychotherapy.* New York: Grune & Stratton.
34. Crawford, H. (1994). Brain dynamics and hypnosis: Attentional and disattentional processes. *Int J Clini and Experi Hypnos, 42,* 4204-232.
35. Haanen, H., et al. (1991). Controlled trial of hypnotherapy in the treatment of refractory fibromyalgia. *J Rheumatol, 18,* 72-75.
36. Kaye, J., et al. (1994). Hypnosis as an aid for tinnitus patients. *Ear, Nose and Throat Journal, 73,* 309-312.
37. Becker, P. (1993). Chronic insomnia: Outcome of hypnotherapeutic intervention in six cases. *Amer J Clin Hypno, 36,* 98-105.
38. Malone, M., & Strube, M. (1988). Meta-analysis of non-medical treatment for chronic pain. *Pain, 334,* 231-234.
39. Kroger, W., & Stainberg, J. (1964). *Childbirth with hypnosis.* New York: Doubleday.

40. Reed, W.; Andresen, G.; & Minagawa, R. (1982). Hypnotic control of anticipatory emesis in patients receiving cancer chemotherapy. *J Consult and Clin Psychol, 50,* 14-19.
41. Spiegel, D., et al. (1989, October). Effect of psychosocial treatment on survival of patients with metastatic breast cancer. *Lancet, 14,* 888-891.
42. Patterson, D., et al. (1992). Hypnosis for the treatment of burn pains. *J Consult and Clin Psychol, 60,* 713-717.

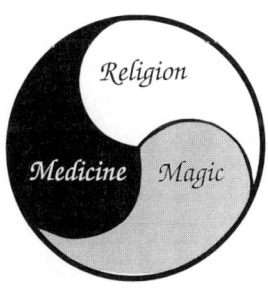

# VI

## HOLISTIC HOKUM AND DOUBTFUL DIAGNOSIS

*"There is no alternative to good medical care."*

IT ALL BEGAN as Voltaire, the Eighteenth Century philosopher said, "when the first knave met the first fool." This truism is supported by many examples throughout the ages.

For hundreds of years, the horn of an imaginary animal — the unicorn — was sold as a remedy for male impotence, epilepsy, worms, smallpox, and other ailments. Since there are no unicorns, walrus tusks, the horn of the rhinoceros, pieces of whalebone and even deer antlers have served instead (1).

In 1635, Rembrandt entitled a drawing with the Dutch word "kwaksalver," referring to a boastful street vendor hawking nostrums. From this came the word "quack." "Quackery" has been defined as the promotion and sale of useless remedies claimed to promote relief from chronic and critical health conditions. The report of the Select Committee on Aging of the House of Representatives, May 31, 1984, stated that quackery reflects pseudoscience at its best. It was pointed out that among persons with chronic illness for whom allopathic medicine has as yet no answers, there will always be the hope for some miraculous cure. There will also always be persons ready and willing to foster that hope. Alternative and cult treatments hold great interest and potential profit for those who wish to practice medicine without the rigors of a scientific medical education. For many, it is not only the patient who believes in the supposed power of an unproven therapy, for many cultists are sincere but naive believers.

The first quack medical device patented in the U.S. was the "mechanical tractor" of Elisha Perkins in 1797. This was said to cure patients by "drawing out bad electricity." In the United States during the late 19th and early 20th Centuries, traveling medicine shows hawked their worthless liniments with widely exaggerated claims. With the discovery of vitamins and the knowledge that rickets and scurvy were due to vitamin deficiency, promoters began to claim that most other illnesses could be cured or avoided by taking vitamin supplements.

Thus began the dawn of what Young (2) calls a nutritional myth that today underlies a mighty health food industry supported by millions of gullible citizens. He estimates modern quackery to be a sophisticated $40 billion business and cautions that if a claim sounds too good to be true, it probably is!

As Sabbagh (3) has pointed out and as we discussed in the chapter on Magic and Mysticism, fringe medicine has much in common with the paranormal. Astrology, palmistry, phrenology, and psychic surgery all crop up in the menu of alternative medicine, depending upon the gullibility of humans for their continued acceptance and financial success. He describes two factors contributing to cures reported by fringe medicine. The first occurs because there is a natural variability in all disease. Hence, at some time in treatment, every patient who does not die will appear to improve in spite of, but not necessarily because of, what is being done. He also calls attention to a second fact, namely, that fringe practitioners rely heavily on placebo responses. In fact, they tend to monopolize the concept of mind/body medicine. They thus completely ignore all the data acquired by research in the field of psychosomatic medicine that occurred in the United States in the early part of this century. They fail to recognize that the beneficial results of fringe therapies can occur because of a belief in the practitioner rather than as a result of any manipulation, preparation, or device. "Unfortunately, negative evidence rarely has an impact on fringe practitioners, who sometimes seem more like priests than doctors, basing their convictions on faith rather than evidence."

### Selling Pseudomedicine

Ever since the dawn of time, humankind has been prone to believe the unbelievable, presume truth where there is no fact, give credence to mysterious causation, and naively trust every charlatan who comes along with an attractive story. That great showman Barnum, said, "A sucker is born every minute." That gives a sufficiently large audience to support generously what I call the "sideshow of Alternative Medicine." That term, by the way, would be more correctly stated as the "sideshow of Alternatives to Medicine," because for persons who are seriously ill there is no alternative to good medical care.

Basic to the selling of any pseudomedical treatment is mindset. If a person is convinced that the treatment will cure, it will probably be effective in relieving symptoms. Mindset, as social psychologists know it, is strongly culturally determined. Just as our religious beliefs are determined by the culture in which we were raised, so what we believe to be the best medicine depends upon cultural exposure. As Joe Jacobs, former head of the OAM, once told us, the Indian Medicine Man's treatment works only for those raised on the reservation.

In the early part of this century, science was on the upswing. Automobiles, aeroplanes, radio, and television became commonplace and it was clear that man would soon walk on the moon. Modern medicine was filled with scientific technological miracles, and antibiotics became the physician's stock in trade. It was common belief that modern medicine would ultimately have the answer to all illnesses. Wherefore then comes the disillusionment that sends one-third of all patients to seek alternative care? Why are health food stores challenging pharmacies with a phenomenal growth rate of 25% a year? Larry Dossey, editor of *Alternative Therapies in Health and Medicine*, states that society's problem with modern medicine is that we are spiritually confused and searching about for meaning in our lives and our illnesses (4). Others have bluntly said that New Age beliefs are strong today because our society is in turmoil.

Due mainly to dramatic improvements in public health and sanitation, life expectancy has doubled and thus many now face the chronic illnesses that come with aging. Although modern medicine has done a great job with acute and infectious disease, it has little but palliation to offer many who suffer chronic disease. Consequently, an increasing number of patients fall prey to the health hucksters who skillfully hawk their wares to the unwary.

Pratkanis (5) has listed the essentials for selling pseudoscience. These principles well apply to the ever-increasing glossy and boastful ads for the products and practices of alternative medicine. First of all, he says one should make the unavailable look good by catering to wishful thinking. "Wouldn't you like to live longer, be free of pain and have a better sex life?" This really attracts attention. Once a potential patient shows an interest, he is ready to become committed. Offer him something like a "sample package of vitamins" or a "free back examination." If, for example, a patient accepts the free examination, some small problem will be found and the patient will be signed up for a series of treatments.

It is important to manufacture a source of credibility. Bogus diplomas are easy to procure. Degrees for some types of holistic healing require only a few weeks of training. Most cults have a well known "guru" or perhaps quote some important authority out of context. Like the old "chain letter" gimmick, self-persuasion is used to turn customers into salespersons. If one finds that the vitamin sample was helpful, he may be easily convinced to become a door-to-door salesperson using his own conviction to enhance sales and thus his bank account and that of the vitamin manufacturer.

Another maneuver is to draw the potential patient into a group, creating a social identity with shared goals and a common enemy. For example, writers on subjects of alternative medicine like to point out in a self-righteous way that the AMA and FDA are "greedy," are protecting the giant profit-making pharmaceutical industry, and thus are "callous" and not really interested in the patient's welfare.

It is possible to divert the righteous wrath of the FDA from an examination of holistic medicine's untested and potentially dangerous products by redirecting the focus to "health freedom," the individual patient's right to choose whatever treatment he wishes (harmful or not!).

Finally, it is useful to use commonplace examples that are readily accepted and require little thought. Such truisms are:

- If everybody agrees, it must be a fact. If it costs more or is rare, it must be more valuable.

- If the message is strong or there are many testimonials, it must be true.

- If it is "natural," it has to be good, for "natural" is better than "manufactured" (even though the chemical structure is identical).

- Appeal to the "goddess within" complex by speaking of the need to invoke spiritual rather than medical treatment methods when the latter may be indicated.
- Use reverence for science by stating, "It is the latest scientific discovery" or, "This treatment is on the cutting edge."

The above tactics are widely used in the selling of New Age products. It is probably important that many New Age healers are persons without medical training. That means they have not learned the necessity of using rigorous scientific methods for evaluation. They are not familiar with the hundreds of illnesses which exist and may have surface resemblance to one another. Nor are they aware of the vagaries of symptoms and possible fallacies of diagnosis. Cultists speak glibly in generalities about "cures by natural means," the power of "the spirit to heal," and indefinable entities like "body energies." Thus, many holistic treatments are based on faith rather than fact, and hence, are not amenable to scientific testing.

A recent study (6) of the attitudes of 572 primary care physicians toward alternative practices indicated considerable variability in knowledge about alternative techniques. In the absence of definitive evaluations of the effectiveness of such techniques, the rule of thumb used by a chiropractic friend of mine might be useful. He says, "if it sounds goofy it probably is goofy."

Reports in newspapers and popular magazines are no reliable guide to the effectiveness of any given treatment. Journalists are not usually skilled in scientific evaluation and are always seeking sensationalism. Thus, even when reported in medical journals, "promising leads" may turn out to lead nowhere. Beware of "initial studies" with small numbers of patients. Wait for larger studies with adequate numbers for sound statistical treatment. See if a placebo control was used. Was the study paid for by a company that could profit from positive results? Was the work done at a respected scientific institution and were references given to preceding or similar studies?

Unfortunately, greed is a universal trait, and the temptation to defraud extends as well to those who propose to treat suffering and disease. The standard formula is to write a book, invest in an herbal or health food company, get on talk shows, become a "guru," and open a bank account.

New Age publications are multiplying and are replete with advertisements for unapproved combinations of herbs and vitamins. The names are reminiscent of patent medicine days: "Women's Tonic," "Sure cure for male impotence," "Elixer of life," etc. Homeopathic remedies are advertised on the radio to naive listeners who are unaware that homeopathy in the U.S. was discarded 50 years ago when it was pointed out that its four basic tenets were entirely without scientific proof.

Major players are Traditional Chinese and Ayurvedic Medicine. The drawing card of the former is ancient acupuncture based on the myth of *meridian* theory. Following President Nixon's visit to China and the ensuing public enthusiasm for things Chinese, acupuncture, advertised as a "cure-all," received great publicity. This opened the door to nonmedical cultists who welcomed the opportunity to profit from the public's widespread desire to try this "mystical treatment from the Orient."

The popularity and spread of acupuncture was buttressed by two important factors that have kept this ancient practice alive and an important Chinese export: culture and politics. Regarding the first, on our trips to China we witnessed children in primary grades being taught to use "acupuncture points" around the eyes to "improve their eyesight." This exercise was carried forward in higher grades. We were also entertained in several schools by children playing the role of "acupuncture doctor." Thus, it became clear that belief in the efficacy of traditional Chinese acupuncture is deeply imbedded in the culture from an early age. What is believed so strongly throughout the nation is ripe for export elsewhere, and from the year 500, acupuncture was exported to other countries around the globe.

In recent years, the role of politics has become important and the Chinese government has looked favorably upon the promotion of overseas markets. China has found a ready market for the sale of acupuncture equipment throughout the world. This was furthered when Chairman Mao, faced with a great need for physicians, promoted the use of "barefoot" doctors and pronounced acupuncture a national treasure. Chou En-lai emphasized that studies must be done using traditional Chinese methods of treatment. The World Health Organization saw that acupuncture worked in China and proclaimed that it could well be the answer to bringing treatment to third-world countries. WHO then encouraged China to develop acupuncture training centers. Such centers for

Traditional Chinese Medicine now flourish and they assist China's profitable tourist industry. China is rightly proud of its past with inventions such as printing, the compass, gunpowder, and others that have spread around the world. In this light, traditional acupuncture with its ancient beginnings is looked upon as another medical innovation. In many countries, naive physicians and thousands of "wannabe" doctors have taken the bait. Promotion in the U.S. has included believers in the mysteries of ear acupuncture. Despite the fact that meta-analysis of the literature (7) has shown this method to be primarily placebo, the unproven method of "needles only" ear acupuncture has been promoted as a treatment for drug addiction, with widespread acceptance throughout the United States. Recently, ancient Chinese medical witchcraft has been resurrected with *Qi Gong* magicians entering the profitable U.S. lecture circuit.

Ayurvedic medicine is simply a newly dressed-up revival of ancient Hindu folk medicine. Along with the usual recommendations for diet, exercise, and meditation is a great variety of bizarre primitive practices using urine, saliva, and purgings. Andrew Skolnick (8) revealed the questionable practices of the Maharishi's multi-billion dollar U.S. Ayurvedic Medicine empire linked to its expensive health salons, recommendation and sale of its own herbal remedies, and advertisements for prophecy and the teaching of *sidhi*, a yogic method in which, for an extra payment, persons are promised to be taught a method by which they will be able to become invisible, walk through walls, and fly. A recent TV program showed one of the Maharishi's lieutenants demonstrating his "miracles of healing" in the setting of his two and a half million dollar mansion. The State of Oregon chastened another Ayurvedic Guru scam whose adherents fled, leaving behind them a stable of Rolls Royce automobiles.

Yes, it's fun to be fooled by magic, but not when that magic involves your health!

**Desirable and Doubtful Diagnostic Procedures**

Hippocrates, father of modern medicine, proclaimed that a careful diagnosis was as important as appropriate prescribing.

What brings the patient to a physician for help? Is it pain? Is it general malaise? Is it a fever or a lump? Whatever it is, the physician must first determine as accurately as possible what is to be treated. The more accurate the diagnosis, the more likely the treatment is to be specific and helpful.

A carefully taken history is the most important diagnostic tool, and of itself may lead to the correct diagnosis. After the history, an examination of the patient is the next important procedure. This, as taught in medical schools, focuses primarily on that part of the body which the history has indicated as the area of trouble or the area to which the patient refers his complaint.

To gain additional information helpful to diagnosis, the physician orders a laboratory examination of body products such as blood, urine, feces, sputum, or specially taken tissues such as a biopsy of a suspected tumor or cerebro-spinal fluid. Other studies may then be indicated, including such non-invasive procedures as X-Ray, EKG, EEG, ultrasound of a particular body region, a CAT scan, or NMRI.

This is the schema of modern diagnostic medicine. This is far and away the best and only sound way to arrive at a conclusion as to what has gone awry with the patient's body. The results achieved by such scientific methods of diagnosis have led to treatments that have saved millions of lives.

Diagnostic procedures pursued by practitioners of alternative medicine had their origin in more primitive times when there was no scientific knowledge of body functions, physiology, chemistry, or anatomy. Therefore, diagnostic methods of alternative medicine may be based either on procedures that are unsupported by facts or on observations cloaked in bizarre, unscientific interpretations. Thus, diagnostic procedures performed by practitioners of alternative medicine may proceed under the supposition that some "body force" is "out of balance." As such "mysterious forces" are simply conjectures, there is no scientific method for measuring them. Thus, the "holistic" practitioner performs a magic ritual and then proceeds with his esoteric treatment. The ritual procedure that is initiated, if the patient believes it, can have placebo value. Should the procedures of the "holistic" practitioner substitute for or delay the proper diagnosis and treatment for an illness with a known specific cure, then that delay could be harmful or life-threatening.

The following are some unscientific methods of diagnosis:

***Shamanic Diagnosis.*** The shaman or medical man is the oldest of healers, the central figure of the primitive religious system which developed in pre-Bronze Age times. Even today in the Arctic, Siberia, the rain forests of South America, and some parts of Africa, a great portion of the world's population relies on the shaman to diagnose and treat illnesses. Derived from the Tunguso-Manchurian word *saman* meaning "he who knows," the shaman is both healer and diviner. By using drums, drugs, dancing, and many bizarre animal and natural artifacts, the shaman enters a trance-like state and claims to travel to the spirit world in order to gain knowledge about the patient's disease. In actuality, the shaman does not leave his body. As a repository of the ancient history of the tribe he/she simply goes into a trance state and recalls ancient bits of wisdom and myths that best fit the healing occasion.

In modern usage, the term "psychic" or "intuitive" diagnosis replaces "shamanic" to describe the supposed powers of persons claiming to have paranormal abilities to use only the mind as the diagnostic tool. As practiced by the spiritists of Sao Paolo, Brazil, a team of "sensitives" is required. Others, on an individual basis (such as Edgar Cayce (9)) fall into a deep sleep and can answer questions seemingly beyond their education and experience.

Some claim to see a colored aura of light surrounding the patient — bright and sparkling in healthy persons, dull and colorless in the sick. In the 1970's, there was considerable excitement over Kirlian photography, in which it was felt that by using an electrostatic photographic technique, an individual's aura could be captured on film. As time went on, a number of experimental artifacts have been described that could account for this seemingly "scientific" diagnostic procedure (10).

In Western U.S.A., some Indian tribes still rely on their medicine men, sand paintings, and tribal dances for both diagnosis and treatment. In primitive areas where modern medicine has not yet become available, such methods are accepted, believed in, and, combined with the tincture of time, may assist the healing process.

***Astrological Diagnosis.*** In early days, medicine and astrology were one. Today, modern practitioners of astrology seek guidance for making their medical diagnoses by examining "cosmological correspondences of the human body." The astrological reading is developed from charts showing the position of planets at the time of the patient's birth. This is the basis of individualistic prescriptions. A biological and medical interpretation is made from the planets and so-called midpoints (Midheaven, Ascendant, Sun, and Moon). Three planetary pairs are the usual combinations for determining disease (Mars/Neptune, Saturn/Neptune, and Sun/Neptune). Astrologers claim that they can be of great help in diagnosis by directing the healer to a particular area of trouble when the case is obscure. Astrologers claim that their approach is holistic, looking at the whole body and promoting wellness through the advice that is given.

Four independent surveys of published predictions found no evidence that astrologers can predict any better than guessing. Seven studies of chart interpretations found no evidence that astrologers can discriminate between right and wrong horoscope charts, suggesting that the perceived validity of astrology is only an illusion (11). Attempts to evaluate astrological readings are confounded because chart interpretations are wordy, rambling, and replete with double meanings. The patient reads into the prediction what he/she wishes to believe is true. For example, taking a single descriptor from the astrological sun-sign and reading from Aries through Pisces one finds as follows: *assertive, possessive, changeable, sensitive, creative, critical, harmonious, secretive, adventurous, cautious, detached,* or *intuitive.* Because we are interested only in our own person, we select the words we feel best fit our opinion of ourselves and ignore the others. Inasmuch as everybody behaves in each of these ways at various times of life, astrology can appear to be true.

Unknown or ignored by most astrologers is the fact that since development of the standard astrological charts many centuries ago, modern astronomical readings are additionally flawed because of the precession of the equinoxes. Thus, traditional astrological charts are in error by nearly a full "house." For example, a person born under the sign of *Pisces* would actually have been born in the house of *Aquarius* and thus (if astrology were scientific, which it is not), have the exact opposite personality traits to those of the astrologer's reading. In the field of medical diagnosis, as for all other aspects of life, astrology is just plain hokum. Believe it at your own risk.

***Diagnosis in Traditional Chinese Medicine.*** Traditional Chinese Medicine approaches the concepts of health and disease from a totally different perspective than Western medicine (12,13). Basic is the concept of polar opposites, *Yin and Yang*, which are believed to be in a constant dynamic state of expansion and contraction. This concept of "energetic medicine" is based on the belief that there is a continuous generation and flow of energy (*ch'i*) through the body over meridian channels. When the flow of these energies is in balance, a condition of health exists. When *Yin* and *Yang* are out of balance, illness occurs.

Each of the 12 major *meridians* is linked to a major organ system. Diagnosis is therefore directed at determining the balance of *Yin and Yang* in the 12 *meridians*, and at deciding what procedures are best used to correct any imbalance that is detected. In the belief that external stressors affect internal organ functioning, the Oriental physician observes carefully the posture, skin color, and eyes. The tone, pitch, and tempo of the voice are evaluated and the patient is questioned carefully regarding diet and life habits.

The method of pulse diagnosis is of prime importance. This is the basic procedure for supposedly detecting energy flow in relation to the twelve body systems. Pulse diagnosis is based on a belief that in a three-centimeter segment of the radial artery at the wrist, one can detect the state of energy in six organ systems on the left hand and six different organ systems on the right hand. The examiner feels first superficially for three organs and then feels deeply for another three at each wrist. Classically, there are 27 varieties of pulse to be distinguished. Hence, the pulse diagnostician is thought by this method to determine not only which organ system is weak or strong, but also the nature of the illness typified by that particular pulse.

From the point of view of practical physics, pulse diagnosis is an impossibility. The pulse at the radial artery is a direct reflection of the strength of the bolus of blood that is ejected by each contraction of the left ventricle of the heart, and nothing more than that. That is the only thing that it is or can be. The fanciful belief that the status of 12 body organs is in some mysterious way superimposed upon this ebb and flow of blood, and that different organ systems are represented on the left and the right is simply metaphysical jargon. Both left and right pulses are derived from the same arch of the aorta and therefore carry an identical beat and rhythm.

If pulse diagnosis must thus be rejected as a physical impossibility, the total structure of a diagnostic system for detecting *Yin/Yang* balance and the selection of points on specific *meridians* for its manipulation are highly questionable.

What, then, is left of value in the Traditional Oriental Medicine diagnostic system is the basis of other primitive systems of diagnosis East and West; that is, the physical examination of the total body. Like other components of alternative medicine, this in turn places a reemphasis on attention to diet and exercise, the proven twin approaches to sound preventive health practices.

***Diagnosis by Iridology.*** The ancient Chaldeans recorded readings of illness from the eye, and observations of the iris in states of disease were reported from Ancient China, Japan, and India. The first designation of iridology as a formal diagnostic method, however, was by the physician Ignatz von Peezely of Hungary in 1868. One day, his pet owl broke a leg, and he noticed soon after a peculiar "rod-like" discoloration in the bird's iris. From this observation, he developed the theory of iridology and published his thesis.

This was followed in 1871 by the appearance of a book on the subject by N. Liljequist, a Swedish minister. In the 1950's, iridology was popularized by American chiropractor Bernard Jensen (14).

Modern iridologists take a color photograph to compare with diagrams indicating circular zones of color and markings that refer to: a) the stomach, b) the intestines, c) blood and lymph systems, d) organs and glands, e) muscles and skeleton, and f) skin and elimination. In general, the upper half of the iris refers to the top half of the body — including brain, neck, lungs, and throat — while the lower half of the iris refers to the lower half of the body. Different degrees of light and darkness, dark marks, and grained patterns are thought to indicate degrees of health and illness.

While allopathic physicians typically examine the eyes for diagnostic purposes, they do so to note action of a reflex of the muscular iris which controls the size of the pupil. In addition, certain patterns around the outer rim are indicative of atherosclerosis or a specific neurological condition, Wilson's disease. The claims of the iridologists that all the body organs are reflected in the iris have not been substantiated, nor do they make anatomical or physiological sense, considering the embryologic development of the iris.

Two double-blind studies of iridology have been made. One involved identifying disease of the gall bladder (15), the other of kidney disease (16). In both instances, the diagnostic ability of the iridologists did not differ from chance. Iridology as a diagnostic method is a hopeful but deluded gleam in the eye of the holistic practitioner.

***Diagnosis in Ayurvedic Medicine.*** Like Traditional Chinese Medicine, the philosophical basis of Ayurvedic medicine is a system of supposed body energies, a balancing of three forces or *doshas* (17). The ancient practice of pulse diagnosis is said to have first originated in India.

Initially, the Ayurvedic physician examines the patient on three different levels in terms of the *tridosha*: air, water and fire. These, in turn, are divided into two aspects, the *purusha*, or physical life and conscious state of man, and the *prakriti*, or subconscious and spirit. The *purusha*, in turn, is divided into three parts:a) self-contentment and rational, b) positive but lacking equilibrium, and c) negative man — on one hand angry, fiery, and impatient and on the other passive, irresolute, and lacking initiative. The physician must first identify these characteristics by observing the patient's attitude and behavior.

The Ayurvedic physician then assesses the *gnanendriyas,* or senses, including sight, touch, taste, smell, hearing, and sex. Next in the examination are the *karmendriyas,* organs controlled by the senses —the tongue, arms, legs, anus, and reproductive organs. The channels or *shrotas* include internally the veins, arteries, lymphatics, intestine, and liver, and externally the eyes, ears, mouth, nostrils, breasts, and vagina. The *manas* include mental desires, lusts, and aversions. The *malas* are the result of man's daily activities — the waste products — urine, feces, and sweat. Finally, the physician's diagnosis takes into account the patient's age, nationality, life, and family circumstances.

From this broad wholistic appraisal, recommendations for treatment are made. These are essentially common prescriptions for good health, including diet, exercise, life style, and herbs and vitamins. These recommendations are accompanied by various mystical and ancient rituals and are at times admixed with medicines from the West.

***Diagnostic Homeopathy***. Homeopathic treatments are individualized and directed wholistically at the total symptom complex of the individual rather than at any disease entity. The homeopathic physician looks at conditions as acute or chronic. In acute conditions, the body is said only to falter but retain the ability to, in time and with the help of homeopathic remedies, regain balance. The homeopathic physician, while treating the acute phase, awaits the appearance of a chronic phase or reoccurrence of a previous acute condition. This is diagnosed as a *miasam,* consistent with whatever type of infection to which the patient was thought to be prone by having an inherited tendency to some disease acquired by a previous ancestor. *Miasams* are classified as psychotic, syphilitic, psoric, canceric, or tuberculinic. As a result of meticulous observation, the particular area of disorder is identified.

In diagnosing, the homeopath takes into account the interdependency of the patient and his/her social, domestic, geographic, and industrial conditions. The character of the patient's mind and temperament, occupation, mode of living, and daily habits are studied. Among items assessed are whether the patient feels better in the morning or evening, whether the right or left side of the body is worse, and items of supposed cosmological significance.

The homeopathic physician thus evaluates the total person, but uses a somewhat individualistic diagnostic approach, guided by the unique aspects of each patient, e.g., his or her mental and physical life, and the particular symptoms that he or she manifests. The specific homeopathic treatment which is then used is tailored not to the disease entity as in allopathic medicine, but to the individual patient as a whole.

When the homeopathic physician is an M.D., D.O., or chiropractor, he may strengthen his diagnostic abilities by using techniques and insights developed from his scientific training.

*Kinesiology and O-Ring Diagnostics.* Kinesiology was invented by the American chiropractor Dr. George Goodhart (18) to assess the energy balance of the body by using a series of muscle-testing procedures applied manually. He felt that relative muscle strength and tone could reveal the energy balance in each of the body systems, stomach, lungs, intestines, etc. He identified the relationship between specific muscle groups and specific body organs. Using this method of muscle testing, he would diagnose disease or compare the effectiveness of various vitamins or food products placed beneath the tongue. Needless to say, this method lacks any scientific validation.

In 1985, Yoshoki Omura, M.D., described a variant of kinesiology called the O-ring test (19). The method of diagnosis is as follows: the patient forms a ring by curving the index finger to touch the tip of the thumb. The testing physician forms a similar finger ring linked to the patient. Then, using the other hand, a wand is moved over the patient's body. Whenever there is perceived a weakening of the strength of the patient's O-ring, the area being touched is presumably a seat of disease. Explanation of this method is derived from Oriental concepts of energy flow and *meridians*. The procedure has become even more fantastic by the use of an intervening *Qi Gong* master acting as an intermediary in the testing procedure (20).

Kinesiology has been shown to be based on suggestion and the patient's psychological state of mind. Since *meridians* do not exist, using that concept to explain the action of the above diagnostic methods is groundless.

*Hair Analysis*. This is based on the assumption that components in hair reflect the general health of the body. Barrett (21) pointed out the fallacy of hair analysis. Samples of hair sent to different laboratories have been given differing analyses.

A patient came to me with a printed analysis of her hair that was ordered by a New Age cultist. Analysis of minerals and other components consisted of over 40 entries. Many were marked as "outside of normal limits." One impossible and frightening entry said the patient was "at risk for Alzheimer's Disease and cancer." On the basis of this, the cultist sold the patient $400 worth of vitamins and herbal preparations, claiming that they would correct the supposed problems.

*Palmistry*. Palm reading is an ancient practice based on a belief that the hand has lines connected to the brain and other organs. Palm readers usually present themselves as "fortune tellers" who prophesy about all kinds of life events, including health and disease.

Several lines on the hand are supposed to be important in forecasting health matters. The Life Line, which circles the thenar eminence, indicates a long or short life according to its length. Various markings on this line indicate times of illness. Similarly, there is a Health Line, running from the base of the fifth digit towards the wrist. Also of supposed important is the Heart Line, spanning an area below the digits from the forefinger to the small digit, and the Head Line, running parallel to and below this Heart Line.

Typical of a cheirologist's health readings are such beliefs as:

- A deep scar on the Heart Line shows danger of apoplexy.
- Fainting fits are likely to occur if the Health Line rises toward the Heart Line.
- Heart disease is indicated if the Heart Line is broken.
- Indigestion is shown by a wavy Health Line.
- Internal troubles are indicated by islands on the Health Line.

Needless to say, these beliefs have no basis in fact. Such diagnostic palmistry is nonsense.

Changes in the overall appearance of the hand, however, can play an important role in any careful physical examination. Berry's book, *The Hand as a Mirror of Systemic Diseases* (22), demonstrates in detail the importance of changes in the hand's structure and appearance in a great number of diseases.

*Psionic Diagnosis, Radionics, Radiesthesia.* Radiesthesia is a method of diagnosing by a process of dowsing (23). The movements of a pendulum held over a sample of hair, blood, saliva, or even a photograph of the patient are noted. The pendulum's motion is interpreted as the diagnosis. In similar manner, the treatment is chosen by finding the same pendulum-swing when held over a number of remedies, usually vials of homeopathic preparations. The principle of radiesthesia is said to be due to a suprasensitive extra-sensory perception by the operator. Psychic emanations from the patient or the patient's effects are believed to influence the swing of the pendulum. Often, an impressive-looking device is used to hold the patient's photograph, fingernail parings, etc., as well as the treatment specimens. This gives the false appearance of a scientific diagnostic procedure.

In Radionics, the diagnostic procedure uses an apparatus claimed to measure electromagnetic vibrations emanating from the patient or even from the patient's body fluids, photograph, etc. The vibrations are then analyzed and identified.

The above diagnostic methods come under the umbrella term "**psionic medicine,**" which is essentially an attempt to resurrect a mystic and magical concept from ancient times. Although aided by a variety of devices, the principle remains the same as that in pre-scientific Egypt and reported in England in 1683. That concept is commonly known as **dowsing** (24). In common non-medical applications, the dowser holds a forked stick of witch hazel in order to determine where to commence digging for wells located over underground streams or objects. Studies have shown that dowsing is most successful in areas where underground streams are plentiful and where dowsers are local persons familiar with the water table distribution.

My first acquaintance with this method was in the form of a "sex detector," purchased from a Johnson-Smith magic catalog. When the bobbin on a string that I received was held over a female hand, it rotated in a circle; over a male, it oscillated back and forth in one plane. I found it to be accurate as long as my mind told me strongly, though subconsciously, the direction in which I wished the pendulum to move.

## REFERENCES

1. *Health quackery*. (1981). Mount Vernon, NY: Consumers Union.
2. Young, H. (1992). *American health quackery*. Princeton, NJ: Princeton University Press.
3. Sabbagh, K. (1985-1986, Winter). The psychopathology of fringe medicine. *Skeptical Inquirer, 10* (2),154-164.
4. Dossey, L. (1995). What does illness mean? *Alternative Medicine, 1* (3), 6-10.
5. Pratkanis, A. (1995). How to sell a pseudoscience. *Skeptical Inquirer, 19*, 19-25.
6. Blumberg, D., et al. (1995). The physician and unconventional medicine. *Alternative Therapies. 1* (3), 31-35.
7. Ter Reit, G.; Kleinjen, J.; & Knipschild, P. (1990). Meta-analysis into the effect of acupuncture on addiction. *Brit J Gen Prac, 40*, 379-382.
8. Skolnick, A. (1992). The Maharishi caper: JAMA hoodwinked (but just for awhile). *Skeptical Inquirer, 16*, 254-259.
9. Carter, M., & McGary, W.I. (1972). *Edgar Cayce on healing.* New York: Paperback Library.

10. Watkins, A., & Bickel, W. (1986). A study of the Kirlian effect. *Skeptical Inquirer, 10,* 244-257.
11. Culver, R., & Ianna, P.(1988). *Astrology: True or false?* Buffalo, NY: Promethius Books.
12. Porkert, M. (1974). *The theoretical foundations of Chinese medicine: Systems of correspondence.* Cambridge, MA: MIT Press.
13. Ulett, G. (1992). *Beyond Yin and Yang: How acupuncture really works.* St. Louis, MO: Warren Green.
14. Jensen, B. (1952). *Science and practice of iridology.* Escondido, CA: Bernard Jensen.
15. Knipschild, P. (1988). Looking for gallbladder disease in the patient's iris. *Brit Med J, 297,* 1576-1581.
16. Simon, A.; Worthen, D.; & Mitas, J. (1979). An evaluation of iridology. *JAMA, 242,* 1385-1388.
17. Strohecker, J. (Exec. ed.) The Burton Goldberg Group. (1994). *Alternative medicine: The definitive guide.* Puyallup, WA: Future Medicine.
18. Goodheart, G., & Schmitt, W. (1978). *Wholistic dimensions in healing.* Garden City, NY: Doubleday.
19. Omura,Y. (1985). A new, simple, non-invasive imaging technique of internal organs and various cancer tissues using extended principles of the "bi-digital O-ring test" without using expensive imaging instruments or exposing the patient to any undesirable radiation. *Acup and Electro-Therapeutics Res Int J, 10,* 255-277.
20. Omura,Y. (1991). Accurate localization of organ representation areas of the tongue, using the bi-digital O-ring test: its clinical application, and re-evaluation of classical oriental tongue diagnosis. *Acup and Electro-Therapeutics Res Int J, 16,* 27-43.
21. Barrett, S. (1985). Commercial hair analysis: science or scam? *JAMA, 254,* 1041-1045.
22. Berry, T. (1963). *The Hand as a mirror of systemic disease.* Philadelphia: F.A. Davis.
23. Tansley, D. (1972). *Radionics and the subtle anatomy of man.* England: Health Science Press.
24. Vogt, E., & Hyman, R. (1979) *Water witching U.S.A.* (2nd ed.). Chicago: University of Chicago Press.

# VII

# COMPREHENSIVE SYSTEMS OF UNCONVENTIONAL MEDICINE

ALTHOUGH the umbrella term "Alternative Medicine" covers dozens of minor healing practices, major systems of alternative medicine include Ayurvedic Medicine, Traditional Chinese Medicine, Chiropractic, and Osteopathy.

**Ayurvedic Medicine** (1,2)

*Ayurveda* is a Sanskrit word meaning the "Laws of Health" (*Ayur* = life, *veda* = knowledge). It is described in one of the four *vedas* or sacred Hindu texts. It forms the basis of the ancient traditional medical practice of India that originated 5,000 years ago. This is considered to be the oldest medical practice based on the body's ability to heal itself. In Ayurveda, the emphasis is on teaching ways of living in order to prevent disease and live a longer, healthier life.

Texts dating before the Christian Era describe not only an extensive list of herbal remedies, but also indicate that Ayurvedic physicians had skills in surgery. They performed not only cosmetic surgery and cataract removal, but removed gall bladders and various tumors as well. In the early Middle Ages, cultural exchanges occurred with other societies including Arabian, Greek, and Egyptian, which produced changes in Ayurvedic practice. At that time, the influence of ancient cosmological beliefs decreased and there was an increased interest in trephination and the use of the sun's rays for healing.

With the sweeping changes that occurred in India during occupation by the British, Ayurvedic practices fell into decline, being practiced mostly in the remote provinces. Since 1945, however, there has been a resurgence of interest with the teaching of the traditional Hindu practices that existed in pre-empire India. Thus, Ayurvedic Medicine is once more an integral part of the medicine of India; only this time, in addition to the primitive and placebo practices of Ayurveda, some of the effective scientific practices that characterize Western medicine have been added.

In Ayurvedic Medicine, body harmony is dependent upon the principle of *tridosha*. Body energy is thought to be created by the interaction of *vata*, air, the *dosha* that produces movement; *kapha*, earth, the stabilizing force of body structure; and *pitta*, fire, associated with heat and digestion. It is *pitta*, the fire, that is believed to transform the *daphic* material substance into a *vatic* or gaseous form that constitutes the energy of life.

There are five *bhutas* of the universe—air, fire, earth, ether, and water. In the Ayurvedic system, the five elements of the universe represent the five elements of the physical body (microcosm). Earth represents the supporting substance, (bone etc.); water represents the vital fluids such as blood and lymph; fire represents the heat generated within the body; air represents the animation and sensation; and ether represents the various networks such as the nervous and circulatory systems. Food is thought to be composed of these five elements; hence, a proper balance of foods includes a representative of each group.

Treatment by Ayurvedic Medicine consists of herbal remedies, diet, exercise, elaborate massage rituals, herbalized steam baths, nasal purging, laxatives, medicated enemas, and oil baths, along with some of the bizarre healing rituals from primitive times. Apart from the use of herbs which can have curative actions, the treatments are primarily ritual, hygienic measures. These are not just prescribed in a general manner; rather, the Ayurvedic physician tailors the selection of proper diet and other treatment elements to the individual patient.

According to Ayurveda, all people can be classified as predominantly *"vata," "kapha,"* or *"pitta."* (Table I) Patients, however, are not always pure types and demonstrate a blend of characteristics. By taking a careful history and observing the patient, the physician determines which of the three *doshas* is predominant, thus indicating the patient's personality type. The diagnostic procedure may also involve an elaborate taking of the pulse, which, as in Chinese sphygmology (probably having its origin in India), is thought to give specific information about the functioning of each individual organ. Similarly, a map of the major body organs is purportedly on the surface of the tongue. This, in some mysterious way, is believed to determine the function of various body organs. Visual examination of body excretions can also be part of the diagnostic work-up.

| **TABLE I** Characteristics of Ayurvedic Body Types ||| 
|---|---|---|
| **VATA (WIND)** | **PITTA (FIRE)** | **KAPHA (MUCUS)** |
| Thin | Medium build | Heavy-set |
| Dry skin | Ruddy skin | Oily skin |
| Hyperactive | Orderly | Slow, graceful |
| Moody | Intense | Relaxed |
| Vivacious | Short-tempered | Slow to anger |
| Random habits | Never misses meals | Eats slowly |
| Imaginative | Intelligent | Affectionate |
| Nervous | Ulcers | Obesity |
| Constipation | Hemorrhoids | Allergy, sinus |
| Enthusiastic | Loving | Tolerant |
| Intuitive | Articulate | Compassionate |
| Cramps | Acne | Cholesterol |
| Anxiety | Perfectionism | Procrastination |

An individual's system is thought to have the tendency to overproduce activity in one or more of the three humors. The physician's task is to eliminate the humoral excesses and to strengthen or normalize the functions of the humors where they are overactive or underactive. As the same three *dosha* types are found in minerals, foods, and natural remedies, choosing the correct herbal remedy and diet follows a prescribed course.

Thus, in treatment, the mucus-predominant person should choose foods, activities, and environmental conditions that would decrease the mucus humor and increase the fire and wind humors. Similar considerations would be made with, of course, different prescriptions for the fire-dominant and wind-dominant personalities.

Unlike procedures in Western medicine in which the patient is the passive recipient of the physician's prescription, the Ayurvedic physician instructs the patient to cooperate in proper behavior both in health and disease. The instructions may involve such items as personal habits, selection of a marital partner, and sexual behavior.

In practice, two Ayurvedas exist: one is practiced when the patient is sick; the other is a preventive type of medicine taught to the patient to practice when s/he is well. Ayurvedic medicine is holistic in nature, dealing in an integrated way with both the body and the mind. Any disturbance in one of the three *doshas*, *vata*, *pitta* or *kapha*, will be reflected at both physical and mental levels. A physical event can affect the mental aspect of that *dosha*, and likewise, a mental event can affect the physical body. This feedback from body to mind and mind to body is different from Western medicine, which has its focus on body symptoms with a simple cause-and-effect relationship.

In Ayurveda, as in other ancient healing practices, the underlying philosophical concepts are interwoven with the religions and ritual characteristics of different regions. Thus, there are several varieties of Ayurvedic medicine, which, although differing in terminology and practice, still retain common philosophical concepts.

As an example of a regional difference, Ayurvedic healing ideas were combined with sorcery to destroy enemies among the ancient sects that lived in Sri Lanka. Similar to voodoo practices, the image of the enemy was scratched on the surface of a melon; this was accompanied by rituals to mislead the enemy.

*Yoga* is closely associated with and part of some Ayurvedic practices. This embraces the concept of integrating mind and body and is both a technique and a philosophy. Yogic methods were described in the *Yoga Sutras* which appeared in the 2nd Century B.C.E. There are now many types of *yoga*. Besides the original *Ashtanga Yoga* described in the *Bhavagad Gita* are: *Karma, Jnana* and *Bahakti Yogas*. Better known are those which have been introduced into the United States: *Hatha, Raja, Tantra* and *Integral Yoga. Yoga* emphasizes exercises, meditation and breathing. *Hatha yoga* stresses the integration of the left and right sides of the body. In one set of exercises, the patient practices breathing alternately with the left and right nostrils. Here it is believed that the sympathetic nervous system is controlled by breathing through the right nostril, the parasympathetic by the left. It is taught that during sleep the right nostril operates and that metabolic fires predominate. Therefore, it is best to sleep on the left side.

Yogic technique emphasizes the importance of the seven *chakras* or energy sources relating to specific parts of the body. The *chakra column* (Figure 1) runs up the center of the body. The lowest *chakra* is earth, represented by a four-petal lotus; the highest — on top of the head — is symbolically an inverted lotus with 1000 petals. *Yoga* exercises are an integral part of Ayurvedic medicine. The ultimate aim of *yoga* is to draw energy from the *chakra* at the lower end of the spine to the topmost *chakra*. At this time one achieves ultimate illumination.

When the Maharishi Mahesh Yogi came to Europe and America in the 1960's, he introduced a modernized version of the ancient teaching of Ayurvedic medicine. This was readily adapted to Western thought. In particular, he recommended the concept of Transcendental Meditation (TM) as a means of coping with the stresses of everyday life. Reportedly, (3) TM instructors, at a price of $1,000, promise to teach *sidihs,* a high state with supernatural powers to become invisible and fly through the air.

As Kurt Butler (4) points out, Ayurvedic medicine is simply ancient Indian folk medicine, consisting of recommendations for good health such as diet, exercise, and relaxation. It recommends many of the medicinal herbs found in old Ayurvedic texts whose safety and effectiveness lack scientific documentation. Ayurvedic medicine resembles other traditional healing practices, but what gives it a unique flavor are the many strange rituals and beliefs admixed with some of India's many religious practices. Butler quotes Ayurveda as claiming that TM practices can reduce crime rates throughout the world. Andrew Skolnick (5) associates some Ayurvedic practitioners with money-making schemes and an attempt to falsely present Ayurveda in a scientific light.

Among the treatments recommended by Ayurvedic healers are not only the use of strange enemas and massage with exotic oils, but also preparations made from animal feces and the patient's own urine and saliva. Claims of cancer cures and the ability of *yogas* to "fly through the air" are linked with grandiose schemes to build expensive homes for "Cities of the Immortals" and cure all the illnesses of the world. The whole is cloaked in an air of mystery that has created a road to financial success for Indian entrepreneurs who have found such magic highly salable to the gullible American public.

# Comprehensive Systems of Unconventional Medicine

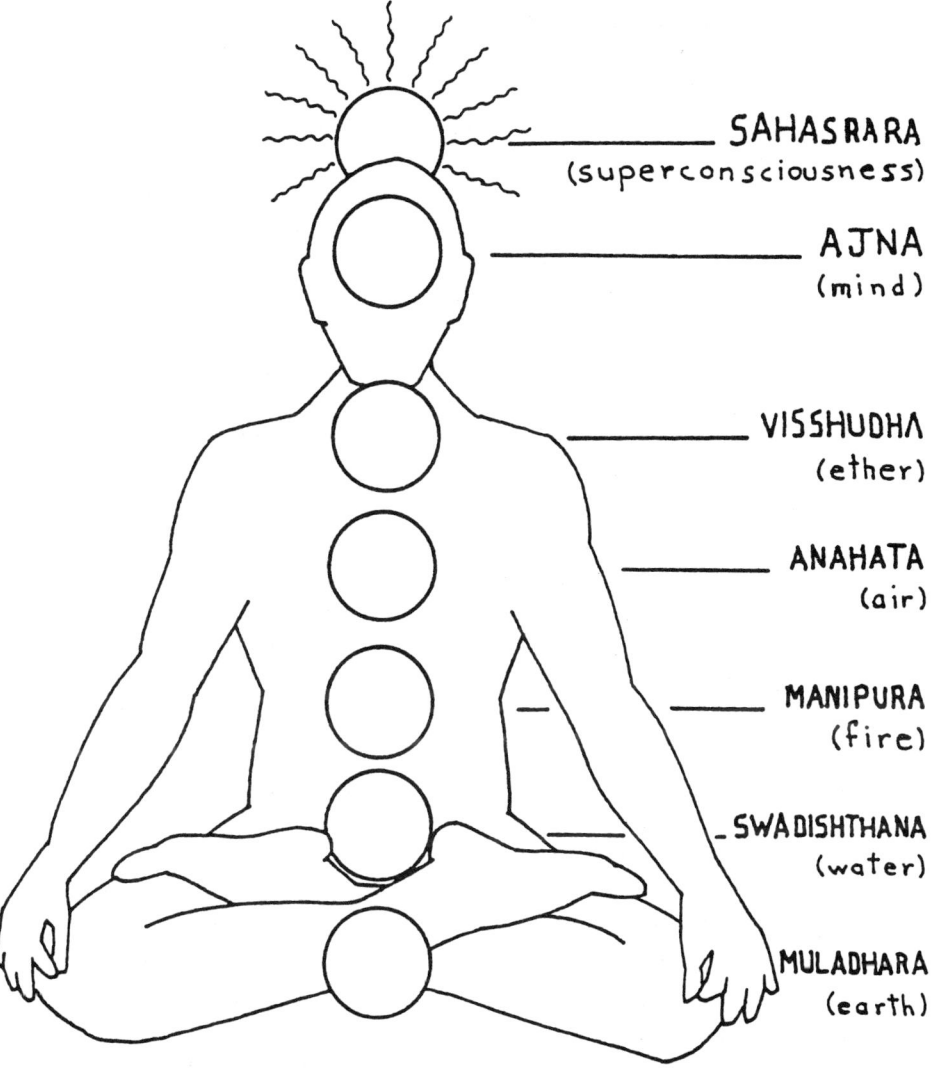

Figure 1. The five elements of fundamental energy forces corrspond to the energy centers of the body.

**Traditional Chinese Medicine**

In classical Chinese medical theory, an energy called *ch'i* is thought to be distributed throughout the body by a series of conduits *(sinarteries)* called **meridians**. Where these *meridians* come near the surface, there are hundreds of points *(hsueh)* or **foraminae** utilized for treatment with needles, finger pressure, or burning of *moxa (artemis vulgaris)*.

*Sinarteriology* is the theory of the energetic conduits *(ching-mo, ching-luo)* with their sensitive points, the *hsueh*. This "*meridian* theory" is the essential ingredient of Chinese medicine, playing a role in diagnostics, pharmacotherapy, massage, acupuncture, and moxibustion.

Modern medicine deals with material structures and tissues which perform certain bodily functions. Classical Chinese medicine (6), on the other hand, deals with functions to which physically demonstrated organs are only incidentally attached. An example is the concept of *san chiao,* translated as "triple heater." It is a vaguely defined area of the central and lower abdomen in which one of the body energies, *ch'i*, is supposedly produced. It is on a par with the eleven other organ systems, each of which has a correspondingly named *meridian*.

Although the medical systems of all great civilizations have had some knowledge of hyperalgesic points or zones, they have nowhere approached the systemic perfection of Chinese *sinarterology*. The origins are lost in the darkness of ancient history, but apparently stone needles were used for the treatment of disease in the second millenium B.C.E. Primitive people at the end of the Stone Age knew that through the stimulation of such points on the surface of the body, illnesses could be influenced. It was not until 300 to 100 years B.C.E. that neighboring points were then diagrammed with lines drawn on the body as though the points were actually connected by conducting channels—the *meridians*. These were then accepted as the main channels for the conduction of *ch'i*.

It is important to note that these sensitive points provided the primary empirical data on which the theory of *sinarteriology* is based. The conduits, or *meridians*, are only the result of speculation. Contemporary physicians in Russia, Japan, China, and the West have tried in vain to prove the existence of such conduits, failing to recognize that their only importance is as an hypothetical construct invented for the support of a metaphysical theory. They are thus analogous to the lines of force drawn on diagrams of a magnetic field or the orbits of planets. The importance of these *meridians* is as mnemonic aids used for diagnosis and treatment. According to Porkert (7), a recognized sinologist, the fundamental empirical constituents of the conduit system are *not* the conduits but rather the points. These forminae are what the archaic founders of acupuncture discovered.

In the metaphysical theory of Traditional Chinese Medicine, there are twelve paired major (cardinal) *meridians*, named after the twelve body systems or "orbs." In addition, there are two unpaired *meridians*, one in the mid-line, posteriorly known as the governing orb, and one located in the mid-line, centrally known as the conception orb. Also, there are the reticular conduits (*lou-mo*), the muscle conduits (*chinghin*), and other pathways for presumed types of body energy.

The *hsueh,* now commonly called "acupuncture points," have in some cases a thermosensitivity or electrical existence demonstrable by measurements on the skin (8). The major useful acupuncture points number around 80. These are such anatomical structures as motor points (neuro-vascular hilae), Golgi tendon organs, and points near major nerve trunks (9,10).

An understanding of classical Chinese medicine depends upon a knowledge of the governing laws and philosophical relationships of *Yin/Yang, the five evolutive phases*, (commonly called five element theory), and the concept of body energy, *ch'i*. This is the energy which is believed to travel to all parts of the body with varying correspondence to the five functional orbs that in turn may or may not be related to the body organs for which they are named. It is to be remembered that these mythical concepts were conceived at a time when there was little knowledge of anatomy and physiology as we understand it today.

*Yin* and *Yang* are concepts of a polarity that exists in all of nature. Together, one *Yin* and one *Yang* make the *tao* or *yinyang*. This is a wholeness, or in terms of the body microcosm, complete health or wellness. *Yang* is a moving, causing, changing, expanding, stabilizing force, while *Yin* is a completing, confirming, reposing, sustaining, and contracting force. When *Yang* increases, *Yin* decreases, and vice versa (Figure 2). *Yin* refers to things female, *Yang* to things male, *Yin* to earth, *Yang* to heaven, *Yin* to right side, *Yang* to left. Other correspondences are shown in Table II.

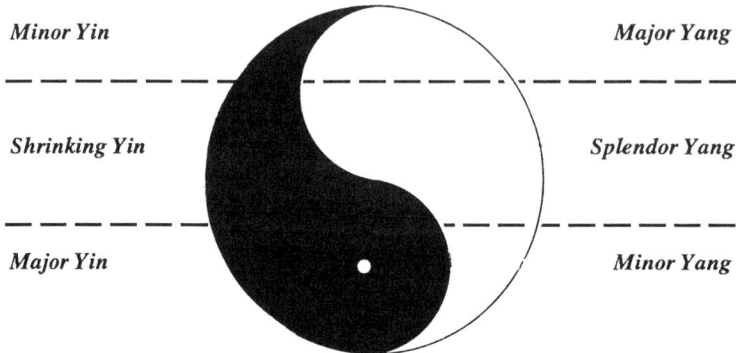

Figure 2. The waxing and waning of *Yin* and *Yang*.

| TABLE II | |
|---|---|
| **PAIRS OF OPPOSITES (*YIN/YANG*)** | |
| **YIN** | **YANG** |
| Earth | Heaven |
| Moon | Sun |
| Winter | Summer |
| Autumn | Spring |
| Female | Male |
| Cold | Hot |
| Inside | Outside |
| Dark | Light |
| Small | Large |
| Weak | Strong |
| Lower | Upper |
| Water | Fire |
| Night | Day |
| Right | Left |

The so-called secondary correspondences are the result of systematizing speculations and relate to changes in *Yin* and *Yang* according to the hours of the day, the inner and outer energy channels of the body, the ebb and flow of energies in regions of the body, seasons of the year, and concepts of astrology and numerology. The strengths and weaknesses of *Yin and Yang* influence such things as diet selection and the 27 characteristic pulses. A universal belief in ancient superstitions plays a significant role in relating the macro-cosm (universe) to the health of the micro-cosm (individual human being).

Early Chinese science and the majority of its basic standards of value were combined into cycles. This was perhaps because they arose in a primitive agrarian society whose very life depended upon the cycles of nature, weather, temperature, generation of crops, birth of animals and the daily and yearly course of the sun and moon.

Second only in importance to *Yin and Yang* in the philosophical basis of Chinese medicine are the **five evolutive phases.** They succeed each other in temporal order (Figure 3). These five phases are combined and intertwined in a seemingly endless fashion. They are standards of value, derived as philosophical and metaphysical concepts, yet constrained as philosophy always is by the scientific knowledge of the day. The basic beliefs underlying the correspondences of Chinese medicine are derived from the cosmic belief in the five elemental substances: wood, fire, earth, metal, and water.

Moving clockwise in Figure 3, the sequence is the evolutive or productive phase. Here, the elements precede one another on the circle. They can also be thought of as having a counter-clockwise ability to check or modify each following element in turn and hence to have the ability to alter the behavior or function of an orb, its related bodily organ. These are known as the *sheng* and *ko* cycles. Disturbances in terms of "deficiencies" or "excesses" may occur through the influence of elements whose position is either strengthened or overpowered by elements connected functionally in the circular diagrammed sequence.

The *sheng/ko* formula indicates how to correct such problems by selecting the proper points on one channel where stimulation can influence the flow of *ch'i* on another channel.

The study of energetic processes of the universe required observations that were based on the fragmentary astronomical data of that time (1,500 years ago), coupled with the rhythms of the sun and moon.

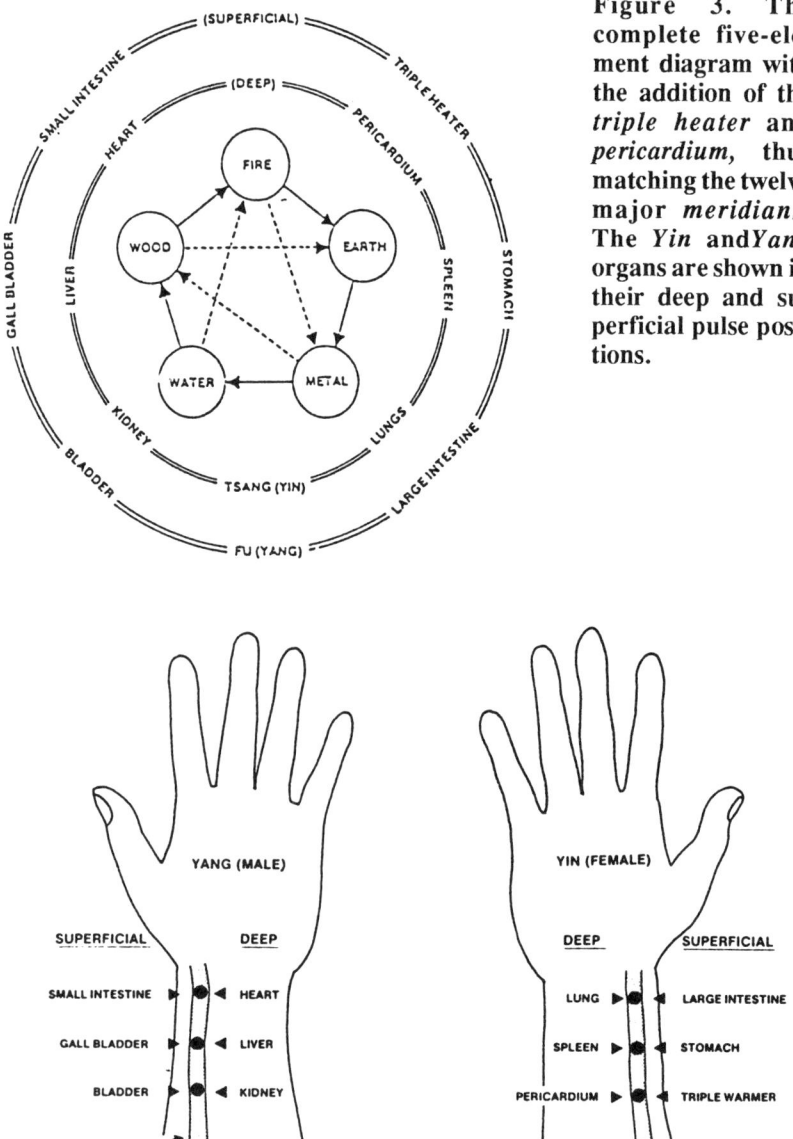

Figure 3. The complete five-element diagram with the addition of the *triple heater* and *pericardium*, thus matching the twelve major *meridians*. The *Yin* and *Yang* organs are shown in their deep and superficial pulse positions.

Figure 4. Location of the twelve pulses in relationship to the energy flow to be detected as reflected from the twelve *meridians*.

The original five evolutive phases became related not to ten, but twelve pulses and twelve major (cardinal) body *meridians*. This came about by the splitting of the fire element (heart, small intestine) so as to include two other orbs, the "triple heater" and the "heart guardian" or pericardium (Figure 3).

These relationships later developed in importance for diagnostic purposes. Thus, the twelve orbs have a relation to: a) body regions; b) sense organs; c) specific body openings; d) psychic-emotions; e) body fluids (urine, blood, sweat); f) actions; g) dream-motifs; and h) anatomical correspondences, the crude speculations and observations of body viscera.

Diagnosis was made by observation of the total body in terms of the above considerations seen in correspondence with the five evolutive phases and their twelve orbs. Pulse diagnosis was a special technique that was used to gain an initial understanding of which organ system required attention. In this, the physician palpated a 3-centimeter segment of the radial artery on each wrist. Six organ systems were thought to be represented on each wrist. Three on each side were felt by superficial palpation and three by deep palpation (Figure 4). At each location, the physician was to distinguish 27 patterns of pulse variation. Once it was discovered which *meridian* system was disturbed, treatment could be directed towards correcting the suspected alteration of energy flow in that orb system by the proper placement and manipulation of the needles.

Treatment was holistic in nature, an approach designed to modify those functions believed to deviate from a balanced *Yin/Yang*. Types of diet, herbs, exercise and modifications of behavior (sex, occupation, etc.) were prescribed in terms of the relationship of the therapeutic agents to the five essences. Specifically, the selection of treatment was made to either "tonify" or "disperse" the deviant functioning orb. The specific treatment method was done in a ritual fashion using needles, herbs, or moxa at the proper body point (*hsueh*).

In Chinese medicine, as in other systems of alternative medicine, is the concept of an underlying life force. In the metaphysics of classical Chinese medicine, the generic term for this force is *ch'i*. More than two dozen forms of *ch'i* are described with specifications of their manner of flow through various of the twelve orbs.

Basic are those forms of energy which travel in the cardinal sinarteries: a) ***Ch'i*** – active. An energy synthesized in the orbis pulmonaris; b) ***Mo*** – an active aspect of the *ch'i* manifested in the pulse as it dynamizes the *hsueh* and induces its circulation; c) ***Ying*** – constructive energy distilled from food within the orbis stomach; and d) ***Hsueh*** – the most profoundly concrete aspect of *ch'i*. The last is more or less equivalent to blood and controlled by the orbis *cardinalis et hepaticus*.

The practical applications of these correspondences are found in the separate disciplines of diagnostics, pathology, acupuncture, pharmacology, and herbology.

Despite its obscure theoretical metaphysical base, Chinese medicine advanced through the ages on a par with and even exceeded some of the advances of medicine in other countries. In the Chien-an periods, about 200 C.E., surgeries included laparotomies, thoracotomies, grafting of organs, intestinal resections, rhinoplasties, and lithotomies. These were said to have been performed under general anesthesia induced by Indian hemp. By the 4th Century C.E., there was some idea of preventive medicine with recommendations for prolonging life by proper diet and exercise. Ko Hung is credited with the first description of smallpox five centuries before the Arabian physician Rhazes. From the 8th Century onward, contracts were signed by fingerprints. Works on ophthalmology, obstetrics, surgery, and pediatrics were available by the 7th Century. Mercury amalgam filling for dental caries was described at that time. Vaccination for smallpox was described in 1014. In the 1700's, missionaries imported ideas of Western medicine to China. However, as late as 1896, soldiers were organized to fire salvos to frighten the demon of the plague. The Boxer Rebellion (1900) signaled a decline in xenophobia and public demonstration of magical cures. Since then, practices of Western medicine have existed side-by-side with barefoot doctors and clinics which still use the metaphysical techniques of Traditional Chinese Medicine.

### Chiropractic

The word "chiropractic" is commonly associated with treatment of back pain, a complaint that most persons experience during their lifetime. It is estimated that 20% of the adult population have low back pain. The usual medical treatments are often unsatisfactory. Of over 200,000 disc operations in the U.S. each year, a conservative estimate shows only 11-15% getting some lasting relief (11). Shekelle and Brook (12) reported that 7.5% of the population made at least one visit to a chiropractor. Of these visits, 42.1% were for back problems and 10.3% for neck problems. Chiropractic, despite growing acceptance since its establishment in 1895, has been the focus of much controversy. Most Americans do not know what chiropractors do. They often fail to realize that chiropractic is a profession and not a type of treatment. Debate in the press regarding the effectiveness, safety, and scientific education of chiropractors reveals a similar lack of information. Even the profession's representatives disagree about some duties and responsibilities of chiropractors. Yet the chiropractic profession is America's largest alternative health care resource.

Chiropractic is a rapidly changing profession. Criticism that you hear may well be of what chiropractic was and not what chiropractic is. Formerly, a method of treatment focused upon a single theoretical basis; chiropractic today is a profession emphasizing hands-on and conservative therapies. Many of the historic criticisms of the profession were well-founded. However, current information shows that old fears about chiropractic are no longer justified. Chiropractic has survived a century of legal battles, professional division, and public debate. The "new" chiropractic profession requires new examination and also new criticisms.

*History.* Like allopathic medicine, chiropractic had its birth pangs in the 19th Century, a time rife with medical and psychic cults. Born in 1845, founder of chiropractic Daniel David Palmer moved in 1886 to Davenport, Iowa, to set up a "magnetic healing" studio. Prior to this, he had been interested in phrenology and spiritualism and in the newly founded technique of osteopathy. Palmer believed in a single cause for all illness. In 1895, he believed his search was rewarded when he restored a patient's hearing by manipulating what he felt to be a misaligned ("subluxed") vertebra in his patient's cervical spine. Palmer was unschooled in anatomy and unaware that the VIII cranial nerve, related to hearing, lies safely confined within the skull and does not reach the vertebral column. Whatever the cause and the cure, Palmer spoke with his pastor of what he had done, and together they coined the term "chiropractic," from the Greek *cheiro* and *praktikos,* "done by hand."

In 1895, he established the Palmer School of Chiropractic with a three-month course. His son, B.J. Palmer, succeeded his father in the school. B.J. had a rugged life, losing his mother when he was less than two years old. He was poorly treated by a succession of five stepmothers. With practically no education, he studied his father's teachings and became a chiropractor at age 16. Unlike his father who died estranged and penniless, B.J. was an extremely successful entrepreneur. Known as the "fountainhead," he was guru of this new cult and died a millionaire. Under his leadership, the training was lengthened to nine months and a mail order course leading to the degree Doctor of Chiropractic was established.

Inspired by his success, other chiropractors rushed to become educators, and it is estimated that at one time, there were over 60 chiropractic schools in the United States. With no regulatory body for standards or curriculum, it is easy to see why chiropractors vary greatly in their knowledge, expertise, and practice. As late as 1945, it was still possible to obtain a mail order chiropractor's degree from a Chicago college. B.J. had no objection to the proliferation of chiropractic schools. He conducted a brisk business in chiropractic equipment, adjustment tables, and books on salesmanship. With his fortune, he travelled the world selling chiropractic and returned to Davenport to build a fine campus replete with art objects from every country in the world. He also became a radio pioneer, establishing in Davenport station WOC ("Wonders of Chiropractic"). To the very last, B.J. affirmed a belief in his father's doctrine that vertebral subluxation was the cause of all disease, and that chiropractors were trained to perform a vertebral adjustment that could cure all disease.

After B.J.'s death, the college was headed by his son, David Daniel Palmer. Under his direction, the curriculum was expanded. By 1970, 22 states required chiropractors to have one or two years of college credit in addition to their chiropractic education.

An early convert to chiropractic was a lawyer in Oklahoma City named William Carver. He established his own chiropractic school a few years after the Palmer school was developed in Davenport. Carver held the view that chiropractors should employ, in addition to chiropractic adjustment, various other methods of treatment, such as physical and nutritional therapy. Palmer disagreed and said that only chiropractic adjustments should be used. This major schism has never healed, and today there are the "straights," who adhere only to Palmer's original doctrine, and the "mixers," who use a varied holistic doctrine.

*Chiropractic Today.* All chiropractors are now licensed by the state in which they practice. The scope of practice may differ according to regulations defined by each state.

Today, there are about 45,000 American doctors of chiropractic. The majority belong to the American Chiropractic Association ("mixers"), with 23,000 members. The other major organization is the International Chiropractic Association ("straights"), which has 6,200 members. There is some overlap in membership and there are other smaller organizations.

Chiropractic is a diverse profession, with 17 schools producing 2,500 doctors per year. The training is broadly founded in both basic and clinical sciences. Apart from chiropractic techniques, the students are taught differential diagnosis and indications for referral. Since 1970, all doctors of chiropractic have been trained according to a set of standards monitored by the profession and the U.S. Department of Education. Today, doctors of chiropractic are required to complete a four-year bachelor of science and doctor of chiropractic program before they may apply for state licensure. Several states require the completion of a four-year degree before applying to the four-year doctorate program.

Although the curriculum is defined by the profession, the content of the classes is left up to the individual schools. The quality of training thus differs considerably among the schools and has fueled diversity, splintering of the profession, volatile discourse, and a hindering of the professions unity. The major schism revolves around the "straights," who support Palmer's original doctrine of subluxation and feel that this, and this alone, is the basic theory and method of their profession. The "mixers," on the other hand, follow the dictum of the American Chiropractic Association, which states:

> Chiropractic practice is the specific adjustment and manipulation of the articulations and adjacent tissues of the body, particularly of the spinal column, for the correction of nerve interference and includes the use of recognized diagnostic methods, as indicated. Patient care is conducted with due regard for environmental, nutritional and

psychotherapeutic factors, as well as first aid, hygiene, sanitation, rehabilitation and related procedures designed to restore or maintain normal nerve function.

The International Chiropractors Association –"straights" – believes:

> The philosophy of chiropractic is based upon the premise that disease or abnormal function is caused by interference with nerve transmission and expression, due to pressure, strain, or tension upon spinal nerves, as a result of bony segments of the vertebral column deviating from their normal juxtaposition. Treatment consists of analysis of any interference with normal nerve transmission and expression and the correction thereof by an adjustment with the hands, of the abnormal deviations of the bony articulations of the vertebral column for the restoration and maintenance of health without the use of drugs or surgery.

With no central regulatory body, a difficult developmental history, and schism in the ranks, the problem of acceptance by other professional disciplines and by the government has been an uphill battle. When the 90th Congress passed the Medicare Act in 1967, the Secretary of HEW named an eight-man expert review panel to advise on the scientific merit of chiropractic and naturopathy. The panel's report at that time recommended against inclusion of chiropractors and naturopaths in the medicare program. Today, however, chiropractors participate in managed care and HMO's.

As their training became more regulated and scientific, chiropractors began to back away from the belief that subluxation is the cause of all diseases. Some, however, continued to claim that manipulation correcting subluxation could cure diseases such as diabetes, asthma, hypertension, and others. However, the very existence of subluxation has been questioned by anatomists and surgeons, including the famous neurosurgeon Dr. Harvey Cushing. In February, 1975, a workshop held at NIH concluded, "...the evidence for the chiropractic subluxation is inferential rather than experimental."

Many chiropractors, recognizing that manipulation was not sufficient to help with the many illnesses with which their patients confronted them, agreed with the "mixers" and added other alternative healing methods to their armamentarium. Prohibited by law from the prescription of drugs or surgical invasion of the body, they adopted such methods as homeopathy, Chinese acupuncture, and iridology. In addition, they became counselors in diet, exercise, and vitamins.

Chiropractors trained in the early days by mail order courses and diploma mills were given more education in salesmanship than in medical ethics. Thus, while malpractice occurs among all healing practices, it has appeared as a particular problem in chiropractic. Due to its unpretentious beginnings, any unfavorable publicity concerning behavioral lapses among chiropractors has produced particularly strong reactions. Criticism has been most severe from the American Medical Association, whose Judicial Council maintained that chiropractic was "an unscientific cult whose practitioners lacked the necessary training and educational background to diagnose and treat human beings (AMA House of Delegates Resolution, December, 1966)." They forbade M.D.'s from all association with chiropractors. Anti-trust suits were then brought by chiropractors against the AMA. These resulted in a ruling by a Federal Court that despite the fact that "...the historic theory of chiropractic, that there is a single cause and cure of disease is wrong...," an injunction was issued forbidding the AMA to engage in any more antichiropractic practices.

Today, chiropractors are licensed to practice in all 50 states. Thirty hospitals in the U.S. admit chiropractors to their hospital staffs. M.D.'s exchange patients with chiropractors, and some teach in chiropractic colleges. In April, 1994, the University of California`–San Diego Medical School held a conference entitled "Cost Conscious Back Care," and invited several chiropractors to participate in the program.

While many chiropractors pride themselves on an holistic approach using a variety of the non-invasive techniques of alternative medicine, the chiropractors who are most acceptable for working with allopathic physicians are those who limit their practice to physical manipulation. Thus, it has been suggested by some that chiropractic should be incorporated within the speciality of physical medicine or physical therapy.

As the concept of subluxation is the very heart of chiropractic theory, the problem for the more scientifically oriented schools is how to define this in keeping with advances in scientific knowledge. Today, for the majority of chiropractors, subluxation is *not* "a bone out of place." Rather, it is thought of as a change in the way somatic tissues react to trauma.

The etiology of the "subluxation complex" is a cascade of events in the tissue surrounding a joint that lead to an inflammatory reaction.

Following the trauma or injury that sets up a barrage of nociceptive or pain impulses, the tissues produce a chemical reaction releasing lactic acid, prostaglandins, leukotrienes, histamine, bradykinen, and others. This inflammatory response aggravates and prolongs the pain and disability. Tension and loss of mobility occur. Anxiety and apprehension, with attendant stimulation of the sympathetic nervous system, induce multiple bodily symptoms and further increase pain. The modern chiropractor views this as the body lesion that s/he hopes to effect through chiropractic hands-on manipulation. The focus is to relieve pain and/or inflammation. Manipulation of the joints and muscles stimulates mechanoreceptors, producing a direct inhibition of the anterolateral system. Relaxation of the muscles occurs through stimulation of gamma-motoneurons and reflex inhibition through the inhibitory interneurons.

*Chiropractic Methods — Diagnosis and Treatment.* Modern chiropractic focuses on strictly structural matters. The chiropractor is a master at handling joints, bones and muscles. Chiropractors are not entirely free of their early heritage, but it is a fact that manipulation can, in an arthritic hand, for example, improve blood circulation, alleviate pain, and improve movement.

After taking a history, the chiropractor performs a physical examination which includes testing the extent of the spine's mobility. The patient may be asked to tilt the head forward and backward and from side to side as the chiropractor tests the dynamics of spinal movement before initiating treatment. Similar testing occurs with the lower spine and, if indicated, the limbs.

Chiropractic manipulations are more properly termed "adjustments." Although there are many variations, most chiropractors rely on manual therapy that can be divided into three large classes.

First is the class of treatments called **High Velocity Low Amplitude Adjusting** (HVLA). In this technique, a quick, shallow thrust is applied to a joint. This moves the joint beyond its usual limit of function. This treatment is designed to reset length sensory organs in muscles, change muscle control of posture and gait, and decrease pain.

Second is the class of treatments called **Low Force**. This is a light, sustained contact in order to mobilize joints. This type of treatment is typically used by members of the osteopathic profession. It is designed to increase circulation in the muscles, produce relaxation, increase range of motion, and rehabilitate muscles by decreasing pain and reducing inflammation.

Third is a class of **Soft Tissue Techniques**. These include deep muscle massage, stretching, and muscle tender point techniques. These are designed to relieve the aggravating reflex muscle spasm that accompanies muscle and ligamentous sprain.

Chiropractic intervention today is often in the role of primary care physicians who treat without the use of drugs. They stress preventive care through nutrition, stress reduction, exercise and life-style changes. Many chiropractors today are interested in sports medicine and industrial injury prevention.

In addition to methods of musculo-skeletal rehabilitation, they use various drugless pain-control techniques. These include such methods as: heat units, cold packs, ultrasound, interferential crossing electromagnetic fields, vibrotherapy devices, whirlpools, pneumatic splints, and other devices common to medical physical therapy.

Nerve stimulation techniques include: transcutaneous electrical neural stimulation (TENS), high-voltage peaked waveforms causing muscle contraction, low-voltage galvanic direct or sinusoidal currents, electro-acupuncture with needles or pads to stimulate the body's natural pain killers, and Russian-style stimulators designed to build strength or exhaust the power in certain muscle groups.

Prominent among the devices found in the chiropractor's office are chiropractic tables. These are specifically selected for the techniques used in the office and are fitted to the doctor's height. Many have moving parts to allow various positions for the patient. The tables may include devices that provide sudden or prolonged stretching, vibration, and heat.

Many chiropractors also utilize diagnostic instruments that are not part of the typical medical work-up. Some of the more rational devices in common use include: postural analyzers, thermal analyzers, gait analyzers, moving x-ray films, roving surface EMG, skin conductivity sensors, and computerized range of motion analyzers. Some of these are experimental in nature.

A large market for gadgets, worthless or of questionable value, comes from the alternative medicine business. M.D.'s, D.O.'s, naturopaths, and others are targets to be duped by this industry. But chiropractors seem to be particularly liable. More than a few opportunistic developers have designed devices and techniques that claim to do what holistic healers would like to do. Such methods include point-finding devices used in auriculotherapy, apparatus, and books extolling unusual forms of acupuncture gadgetry, O-Ring therapy, radiasthesia, iris diagnosis, and others.

*What Chiropractic Actually Accomplishes.* Chiropractic treatment relieves stress from joints and muscles and can decrease pain. Reduction of stress on joints can reduce inflammation and speed healing. Manipulation can have an effect on back and neck pain caused by trauma from work-related and traffic accident injuries. Manual treatments can relieve headaches caused by muscle strain and, in the long run, the regeneration of damaged joints may prevent degeneration caused by immobilization. Because chiropractors do not use drugs, their therapies do not offer a direct cure for most diseases but are rather aimed at methods to enhance healing.

There is much literature criticizing the safety of manual therapy. But today's chiropractors are taught to be well aware of the potential dangers of some types of manual therapy. Malpractice and misdiagnosis is unacceptable in any profession. Because chiropractic treatment is conservative and non-invasive, it holds less chance to cause side effects of major disability or death. The malpractice insurance rates for chiropractors is the lowest of all health care providers, including veterinarians.

More greatly criticized is the chiropractor's use of such far-out measures as clinical kinesiology, neuro-linguistic programming, bio-energetic synchronization techniques, *meridian* theory acupuncture, and other questionable procedures.

*Acceptance of Chiropractic.* Mark Sanders, D.C., a chiropractor who did ten years of private practice, served as an instructor and clinician at a national chiropractic college, and is now concerned with measuring quality control for third-party payers, has reported as follows:

> ...spinal manipulation is an important, bona fide therapy for selected patients, with back, muscle, and nerve problems. I also believe there are many good chiropractors. They practice rationally, attend postgraduate courses, and read medical and chiropractic journals. But others don't, and that hurts the profession. We need to improve our image—and patient care—by further documenting the efficacy of what we do and standardizing our services.

Dr. Sanders reported in *Medical Economics* after doing utilization reviews of the practices of individual chiropractors over a three-year period. He warns against the failure to refer for the proper treatment of medical conditions while a continuation of chiropractic treatments can delay allopathic care for life-threatening conditions. He also warns against manipulation when X-rays indicate that bony malformations of the spine could produce permanent spinal cord damages.

Spinal manipulation is the most frequently employed conservative treatment for low back pain in the United States. Its greatest value is as a first treatment approach in this medical climate where surgical interventions are too often overused and with poor outcomes. The most authoritative analysis of the evidence on spinal manipulation is the *Rand Corporation Literature Review* (13). Its conclusions are based on a review of 74 research sources and 21 controlled trials of chiropractic adjustment and other types of manipulation. The conclusion of the panel is that acute and sub-acute mechanical low back pain treated by spinal manipulation is more beneficial than standard medical management, i.e., bed rest, medication, and traction.

A recent government-funded study group of 23 experts was chaired by Dr. S.J. Biggs, professor of orthopedic surgery at the University of Washington, Seattle, School of Medicine. Their report stated that for most sufferers of low back pain, the problems will go away on their own within a month. Their recommendations frown on surgery, X-rays, CT scans, and magnetic resonance imaging. They dismiss as unproven treatments such as spinal traction, biofeedback, TENS, acupuncture, steroids and injections. But they say that spinal manipulation, usually performed by a chiropractor, "can be helpful for patients with acute low back problems...within the first month of symptoms."(14)

Modern chiropractic thus has the opportunity to play a more significant role in health care today. It is only unfortunate that, despite increasingly scientific training, the continued obeisance to outdated metaphysical beliefs and practices lingers.

## Osteopathy

Osteopathy, from the Greek *osteo* (bone) and *pathos* (disease), originated from the concept that biomechanical dysfunctions of bone, joints and muscle can interfere with circulatory and nervous functioning and thus impair the body's ability to heal. This practice of medicine was founded in 1874 by Andrew Taylor Still (1828-1917), a Civil War physician who received his medical training at the College of Physicians and Surgeons in Kansas City. Still practiced in the tradition of the "bone breakers" of the late Middle Ages, breaking up adhesions and setting fractures. He was unhappy with the crude treatments of his day, i.e., bloodletting, cupping, and purging. His belief that there were ways to strengthen the body's inherent methods of healing itself was intensified through grief when three of his sons died of spinal meningitis.

Still concluded "It is our natures that are the physicians of our disease," and that "Order and health are universally one, in union." Osteopathic medicine is the practical application of these beliefs to the treatment of disease. On this basis, Still founded the first College of Osteopathy in Kirksville, Missouri in 1894 and the American Osteopathic Association in 1897. Although it is today one of the most accepted methods of Alternative Medicine, it was for many years rejected by the orthodox medical community, who felt its training was inferior. Beginning in the 1930's, there was an upgrading of D.O. training. With the shortage of medical personnel during World War II, osteopaths were taken into the army as military officers with status equivalent to M.D.'s. Today, there are over 15,000 osteopathic physicians with licensure in all 50 States. Graduated from any of twelve colleges, D.O.'s practice in over 60 osteopathic hospitals. Osteopaths practice not only their own particular brand of medicine, but have increasingly incorporated the principles and practices of allopaths and are now admitted to the staffs of many allopathic medical hospitals throughout the world.

***The Nature of Osteopathic Medicine.*** In keeping with Dr. Still's concept that the body acts as an integrated whole in which structure and function are completely interdependent, D.O.'s practice a wholistic type of medicine. The osteopath believes that through an understanding of the structure of the human body, s/he can so influence it that normal functioning will return. Dr. Still believed that "the rule of the artery is supreme" and that when circulation could be returned to normal, healing and normal function would return.

Osteopaths do not deny the "germ theory," but stress the importance of correcting the "osteopathic lesion" so that the body's ability to fight disease will be strengthened. Through manipulation, they relieve stresses in the neuromusculo-skeletal system (bones, muscles, tendons, fibrous tissues, nerves, spinal column, and brain) so that the flow of blood, lymph, and nerve transmission can return to normal, giving free access to components of the immune system to the involved area in order for cells and enzymes to enhance the healing process.

The osteopath is concerned with mobility of body parts, such as the rib cage in respiration, etc. Like the chiropractor, the osteopath centers much attention upon the vertebral column. It is felt that with too great a movement or torque upon the vertebral column, the small joints of the individual vertebral bodies will wedge and lock and that the ensuing muscle spasm will press upon the exiting spinal nerves and produce physiological abnormalities. Local inflammatory changes around the injured joint can influence the autonomic nervous system which is responsible for controlling the function of blood vessels, glands, and organs. Hence, distant pathology can develop. In turn, local body pathology can send messages back and thus further disrupt the local function of the spinal cord. Prolonged or more serious afflictions can result in problems with the vertebral discs and, in the long term, spondylosis (spinal osteoarthritis) can develop.

***Examination and Treatment.*** After taking a careful history that includes not only past illnesses and accidents but also an evaluation of life style and stress factors, the osteopathic physician proceeds to the examination. This may include laboratory and x-ray procedures. During the initial examination, the osteopath watches the patient's posture and gait, noting any differences in leg length, shoulder height, and curvature of the spine.

With the patient lying on a couch on his back, the body is lightly palpated for areas of tenderness, swelling, inflammation and muscle stiffness. Each joint is moved through its range of motion using the arms and legs as levers. (This differs from the chiropractic maneuver which is a direct thrust on the vertebrae with the patient lying face down). The patient is taken through a movement that will open the joint with generally a loud click as the joint fluid changes state momentarily with the negative pressure produced. Separation of the joint surfaces allows the structures to glide immediately back into motion, relieving the vicious cycle which maintains the muscle spasm and local inflammation. Occasionally, the D.O. will use a more forceful manipulation of the joint called the high velocity thrust.

In addition to using antibiotics and other medications where indicated, the osteopathic physician will pay attention to diet, prescribe vitamins, and recommend exercise programs. The treatment may be combined with stretching and strengthening exercises designed to improve the circulation of blood and lymph. The patient may be taught relaxation techniques with meditation and breathing exercises designed to help overcome stress.

*Summary.* Osteopathy is the most widely accepted of the techniques of alternative medicine. As osteopaths incorporate more of the techniques of allopathic medicine into their practice, there is a danger that they will neglect some of the important holistic concepts and the manipulation that has been characteristic of their profession. On the other hand, the possibility exists that their association with M.D.'s may bring the latter to a more holistic approach to medical care.

**Sideshows of Alternative Medicine**

The array of alternative treatments is growing by leaps and bounds. There is a phantasmagoria of systems and methods. It is like a great garage sale or a carnival. "You pays your money and you gets your choice!" In reality you get what you believe in. No treatments are specific for your illness. They are generic in nature and advertised to "detoxify," "to balance," "boost your immune system," and "correct your body energy." None are guaranteed to cure and some may actually harm. They may well delay proper treatment and cure.

Jack Raso said it well:

> Alternative health care is a "melting pot" of religion, occultism, folklore, parapsychology, pop psychology, pseudoscience, and medical guesswork. It overflows with theoretical rubbish. In the sprawling, animistic 'enchanted forest' of medical alternativism, ideas run hog-wild, words have magical power, illness ("disease") is an educational opportunity, the impossible is a challenge, wishful thinking is industry, faith is the ticket, and death is a transition. (15)

A sampling of the many methods of Alternative Medicine is listed below.

*Aromatherapy.* This is considered by some to be a branch of herbal medicine. Essential oils extracted from plants are used for the treatment of infectious and skin disorders (16). A few drops of eucalyptus, cinnamon, thyme, melissa, pine, or lavender added to a bowl of steaming water may be inhaled several times a day to treat sinusitis or bronchitis. The skin absorbs oils quickly so that oil rubs of juniper, rosemary, clove, thyme, and olive oil can be used to ease muscle pain or arthritis.

Aromatherapy undoubtedly has a placebo effect with its enthusiastic "therapists" and their rituals. It is not a substitute for proper therapy for the treatment of serious illnesses.

The effects of fragrances on emotions has a long history. The powerful effects of odors are found throughout the kingdom of living creatures. Pheromones, scents that attract creatures of the opposite sex, are ubiquitous. The perfume industry has made use of this characteristic with not-so-subtle advertising.

Like other mammals, humans can detect hundreds of different odors. An infant finds the mother's nipple through the sense of odor and a mother can, in turn, pick out her newborn based on its scent alone. Receptors on the nasal mucous membrane receive molecules of the odorous substance. The receptor cell changes shape and sends a message inward along nerves to the olfactory bulb. These impulses ultimately reach the limbic system of the brain which is the seat of memory, emotion, and sexual arousal.

Memory is a complex phenomenon involving networks of nerves arising from various sensory centers of the brain. One sensation alone, such as a familiar odor, is sufficient to invoke the image and memory of a past experience complete with the attendant emotion.

Aromatherapy is widely practiced in Europe. Pharmacies in France and Germany may stock standard items. The following list includes examples with commonly suggested uses:

> Eucalyptus (antiviral and expectorant)
> Everlast (anti-injury, swellings and scars)
> Geranium (antifungal)
> Lavender (burns and insect bites)
> Mandarin (calming properties)
> Nisouli (oily skin)
> Palmarosa (herpes)

Peppermint (nausea)
Chamomile (stress)
Rosemary (skin care)
Tea Tree (wound healing, mild infections)

Newer applications for aromatics include fragrant sprays for home use, fragrances in stores to entice customers to purchase, and odors that have been shown to stimulate workers to greater production.

***Bach Flower Remedies.*** Edward Bach (1886-1925) was a British physician who, unhappy as a medical student, felt his own intuition was superior to book knowledge. He gave up conventional medicine to study homeopathy. He felt that he could intuit the effects of ingesting a flower simply by holding his hand over it. His eccentricities included the belief that heart disease is caused by the failure to develop love for humanity and that bathing in hot water opens the skin and allows dirt to flow inside the body.

In the late 1920's, he became convinced that dew warmed by the sun absorbs the healing powers from plants. Bach spent the remaining years of his life identifying plants that he felt were capable of changing human behavior. He limited these to 38 because these were the only varieties found around his home.

His familiarity with homeopathy led him to his own variety of the "doctrine of signatures" implying that "like heals like." In his theory, the flower *impatiens* is prescribed for persons who are impatient, *rock rose* is used for those who wish to be strong, *water violet is* given to those who are bashful (the shrinking violet type), while *wild oat is* used for the unconventional who "sow their wild oats." (17)

Since Bach's death, his system has been taken over by others, including manufacturers of aromatics and other herbs. They have expanded the number of plants used and furnish elaborate personality questionnaires, the answers to which describe a person's personality type, and hence indicate the flower remedy to be used. Such recommendations are supported only by anecdotal evidence.

The method of preparing the remedies remains much the same. The flowers are placed in glass bowls filled with water. These are left sitting in the sun for three hours. At the end of that time, the flowers are discarded. The remaining water is believed to have absorbed the healing properties of the flower. This is then preserved in brandy known as the Mother Tincture. Extracts are made from this.

Bach rejected science and believed that all illnesses derived from the qualities of personality. He felt that his flower remedies, by treating personality quirks and emotional problems, would ultimately bring about a cure of various physical disease conditions. It is interesting that although his beliefs were metaphysical and his treatments have questionable value, his theories about the nature of disease have some resemblance to modern thinking about neuro-psycho-immunology, a science that links emotions and health.

*Bodywork.* The term "bodywork" is used in alternative medicine to cover a number of treatment methods including massage, deep tissue manipulation, postural exercises, and several procedures based on a belief that touching may somehow balance theorized "body energies." Some of the more widely known follow.

### Therapeutic Massage

For centuries, muscle spasm, tension, pain, and tissue swelling have been relieved by therapeutic massage. Movement of the hands giving deep pressure and friction can stimulate blood flow and affect physiological functions. There are hundreds of techniques and schools of massage, including Swedish, Japanese, and others. Some techniques as listed below are named after individuals who have incorporated their own ideas and added specific postures, exercises and psychological interventions (18).

#### THE ALEXANDER TECHNIQUE

Developed by the actor F. Matthias Alexander, who felt his voice loss was due to bad posture. He recommended physical education to improve body posture to relieve body tensions and promote health. It is used to improve body functions and relieve pain (19).

#### FELDENKRAIS METHOD

A method developed by the French physicist Moshe Feldenkrais. It combines gentle touch with body training and verbal dialogue to help relieve stress and chronic pain and to train for improved athletic coordination (20).

#### ROLFING

Extremely deep massage to soften chronically tight connective tissue, thus promoting body relaxation and relief from tension. It was developed by a biochemist, Ida Rolf, who was familiar with *Hatha yoga* and had, as a young girl, been treated by an osteopath who repositioned a rib which had caused her respiratory problems. Exercises termed "Movement Integration" stress correction of posture and wider range of muscle movements to improve health (21).

### HELLERWORK

A technique of deep-tissue muscle therapy, movement reduction, and dialogue about emotional issues that may underlie postural strains. Developed by former aerospace engineer Joseph Heller (22).

### TRAGER APPROACH

Developed by Milton Trager, M.D., this is a body awareness technique in which the practitioner cradles and moves the patient's limbs to retrain normal patterns of movement (23).

### REFLEXOLOGY

Treatment using pressure on areas of the feet, which are thought to relate to specific body parts and organs. Evolved from the earlier European practice of **Zone Therapy**, which utilizes massage of the hands and feet to stimulate hypothesized horizontal and vertical body zones that are supposed to relate to specific body organs (24).

### ACUPRESSURE

The use of finger pressure on the traditional points of Chinese acupuncture. Such pressure is supposed to release energy (*ch'i*) blockages on the hypothetical *meridian* pathways. In China it is known as *Tui Na*. In Japan are several varieties known as *Amma*, *Shiatsu*, *Jin Shin Jyutsu*, etc. (25).

### POLARITY THERAPY

Developed by Randolph Stone, D.C., D.O., N.D., from a belief that there are electromagnetic currents in the human body. This is patterned after Eastern concepts of blockages in energy flow which result in illness. The method consists of using pressure points, altered breathing, hydrotherapy, reflexology, and other manipulative techniques with healing resulting from stimulating changes in the electrical polarity of the body (26).

### THERAPEUTIC TOUCH

A treatment based on the belief that illness is caused by a deficiency or imbalance of body energies. A variant of "hands on" healing named and promoted by the nurse Delores Kreiger. The therapist uses the hands to assess the patient's body state of health and to direct energy from the healer to the patient (27). An earlier concept, *Reiki*, is an ancient Tibetan healing system designed to channel healing energies from the hands of the healer to the patient. It was described in an ancient Sanskrit manuscript by a Japanese theologian, Dr. Mikao Usui, in the 1800's.

### CRANIO-SACRAL THERAPY

Manipulation of the bones of the skull in order to treat supposed blockages of the flow of cerebro-spinal-fluid (CSF). Subtle pulsations of the CSF, said to occur with a rhythm of 6-10 cycles per minute, are detected through palpation at the cranial sutures. Sutherland (28), a D.O. who popularized this technique in the early 20th Century, postulated that the bones of the skull are mobile. This is not a fact accepted by anatomists except in infants. He used manipulation in order to affect the pressure of the CSF and thus its effect on the brain and nerves exiting from the skull. Other workers used this technique in the belief that they could alter tension of the meninges or affect nerve endings in the scalp or between the cranial sutures. The theory was broadened to speculate on a relationship between these techniques and various body organs. It is used to treat a variety of diseases, including infections.

### APPLIED KINESIOLOGY

This term and methodology was introduced in 1964 by chiropractor George Goodheart. (29) It is his theory that most muscle spasm is not primary but secondary to weakness of an antagonist muscle. Muscle spasm can produce painful "trigger points" as a result of motor neuron facilitation. Through muscle testing, he demonstrates specific weaknesses which he relates to vitamin and mineral deficiencies, tested by placing the suspected substance on the tongue and re-testing the muscle to see if it has thus regained strength. Later, he incorporated ideas from Traditional Chinese Medicine, "energy fields," and allergy. The technique is used to improve athletic performance and treat athletic injuries. Kinesiologists believe that muscle weakness can indicate problems in underlying body organs, e.g., deltoid weakness relates to lung problems. The effectiveness of kinesiology is supported primarily by anecdotal case reports rather than replicable scientific studies.

**Other Methods.**

### T'ai Chi C'huan

A series of physical exercises and meditation with the aim of reestablishing "the connection between life energy in the universe and life energy in the human being." The movements are slow and stress training in balance, which is particularly good for older patients. This is part of the series of training in Chinese martial arts and closely related to *Chi Kunq (Chi Gonq, Qi Gonq)*, which has both an internal form, stressing breathing and meditation and an external form, in which the master supposedly projects healing energy from his body to a patient.

### Laserpuncture
Application of a laser beam to acupuncture points. The laser used is often weak, and there are no proven healing effects.

### Sonopuncture
Like the above. Applies ultrasound to classical acupuncture points.

### Colorpuncture
Belief that color is "life energy" that carries "healing information." Treatment is with a penlight-type device that shows a spot of colored light upon acupuncture points on the skin.

### Scalp Acupuncture
Places needles in the scalp over areas of the brain believed to control various body functions.

### Karuna Reiki
A method of treatment by "laying on of hands." Formerly known as *Sai Baba Reiki.* It is believed that the therapists channel "universal life energy power" through their bodies and in the solar plexus of "diseased" persons for "rebalancing."

### Ho'opono Pono
Ancient Hawaiian healing method designed for "self discovery" and spiritual "cleansing" and "balance." Can be applied to "any person, problem or object."

### Vibrational Healing (Energy Medicine)
The belief that humans are a "dynamic energy system" that is responsible for health and illness. The system coordinates the "life force" and the "physical body." Treatment includes such methods as: crystal therapy, acupuncture, homeopathy, laying on of hands, EAV (electroacupuncture according to Voll), moxibustion, laserpuncture, and a host of others.

### Reichian Therapy
Wilhelm Reich, an Austrian psychoanalyst, was born in 1897. He began his career as a pupil of Sigmund Freud and spent the years 1922–1928 as Freud's assistant at the Vienna Psychoanalytic Polyclinic. He broke with Freud over his controversial ideas that related neurosis to a physiological basis. His book, *Character Analysis* (30), describes how repressed emotions create chronic muscular tensions, which he termed body "armoring."

He felt that repressed sexual energy could be released through the convulsive-like movements of an orgasm. While working in Oslo in 1939, Reich believed he had discovered a new form of energy, which he called "orgone energy." This, he said, was a form of "life energy," which responded directly to the radiations of atmospheric energy. He believed this could be collected by means of a special "orgone accumulator." This was essentially a wooden cabinet lined with alternate layers of organic and non-organic material such as glass and steel wool. The box was open at the top. The patient stood inside the box in order to receive healing from the "streaming rays of atmospheric energy."

Reich moved to the United States in 1939 to devote himself to his work with orgone energy. He used this as a curative method for all types of illness, including not only mental problems, but even cancer. He was criticized for the basically sexual tone of his work. In 1954, he was arrested for mailing orgone boxes across state lines. He died in a Pennsylvania penitentiary in 1957, a tired and bitter man.

The above list is only a sampling of the dozens of alternative healing systems available. Also, hundreds of books are now sold to the public, advertising various techniques of holistic healing. The titles include many of the New Age buzz-words and phrases that are used to entice the prospective buyer of the book and to become a potential user of the method described. Supportive evidence is mostly anecdotal.

### Treatment — Allopathic and Alternative

Listed below are some common illnesses and their contrasting treatments as recommended by allopathic physicians and by practitioners of alternative medicine. These are not always distinctly separate treatment approaches, but may be used in a combined and complementary fashion. This is especially so when administered by allopathic physicians who have an interest in holistic medicine. The recommendations of alternative therapy are directed primarily at prevention and enhancing the body's own healing abilities. Allopathic treatments, on the other hand, are usually directed toward attacking the causative agent, as in antibiotic therapy, correcting hormonal imbalances, or surgically removing the offending agent.

These treatments are given only as illustrations.* All treatments, allopathic or alternative, should be given only with the advice and supervision of a qualified physician.

## ARTHRITIS

| Allopathic | Alternative |
|---|---|
| **NSAIDS:**<br>　Indomethacin (Indocin)<br>　Naproxen (Naprosin)<br>　Piroxicam (Feldene) | **Vitamins and Minerals**<br>**Anti-oxidant supplements**<br>**Diet:** avoid nightshade foods, check food allergies<br>For *osteoarthritis* **use:**<br>　Glucosamine sulfate 500 mg t.i.d.<br>For *rheumatoid arthritis* **use:**<br>　EPA (eicosapentaenoic acid) – 1-2 gm daily<br>　Bromelain – 500 mg. t.i.d.<br>　Curcumin – 400 mg. t.i.d. |

## ANXIETY—INSOMNIA

| Allopathic | Alternative |
|---|---|
| Benzodiazepenes<br>Antihistamines | **Sleep hygiene behavior**<br>**Valerian:** dried root – 1-2 gm; fluid extract – 1/2-1 tsp.<br>**L-tryptophan:** 1-2 gm<br>**Vitamin E:** 400 mg<br>**Folic acid:** 35-60 mg |

*Adapted from Murray, M. 1994. *Natural Alternatives to Over the Counter and Prescription Drugs.* New York: Wm. Morrow.

## ASTHMA—HAY FEVER

### ALLOPATHIC

**Antihistamines:** Benadryl, Dimetapp, Seldane, Hismanal
**Broncho-dilators:** Alupent, Ventoline, etc.
**Xanthine Preparations (Theophylline):** Theodur, Slo-bid
**Corticosteroids:** Vanceril, Beconase, etc.
**Desensitization injections**

### ALTERNATIVE

**Control environmental pollutants:** pollens, dust, fumes, etc.
**Diet:** avoid food allergens; follow vegetable diet
**Vitamins/minerals:** C, B6, E, selenium, B12 – 1,000 ug I.M.
**Flavonoids:** 250-500 mg just before meals
**Ephedra sinica** 500-1,000 mg
**Quercetin**

## HYPERTENSION

### ALLOPATHIC

**Diuretics:** Thiazide (Diuril, Esidrix, etc.); Loop (Lasix, etc.); Potassium sparing (Aldactone, etc.)
**Beta blockers:** Tenormin, Inderal, etc.
**Calcium channel blockers:** Cardiazam, procardia, etc.
**Angiotensin-converting enzyme (ACE inhibitor):** Vasotec, Capoten, etc.

### ALTERNATIVE

**Diet:** obesity, low sodium, high potassium
**Omega-3 fatty acids:** fish oil (EPA), linoleic (flaxseed oil)
**Life-style change:** avoid stress, caffeine, tobacco, alcohol, heavy meals
**Vitamins/minerals:** C – 1-2 gm; calcium – 1-2 gm; magnesium – 1-2 gm
**Hawthorne:** 100-300 mg t.i.d.

## COMMON COLD

| ALLOPATHIC | ALTERNATIVE |
|---|---|
| Antibiotics | Rest |
| Antihistamines | **High fluid intake:** vegetable juice, herbal tea, soup |
| Nasal decongestants | **Limit sugar and fruits** |
| Cough suppressants | **Menthol preparations:** rubs and balms |
| Expectorants | **Echinacea:** tincture – 1/2-1 tsp. in water t.i.d. |
| ASA | **Goldenseal:** dried root or tea – 1-2 gm |
| | **Glycyrrhiza: (licorice)** dried root or tea 1-2 gm |
| | **Astragalus:** root or tea |

## DIABETES

| ALLOPATHIC | ALTERNATIVE |
|---|---|
| Insulin | **Change life-style:** lower body weight, exercise |
| Oral Hypoglycemics: Diabinase, Orinase, etc. | **Vitamins/minerals:** C – 2 gm; chromium – 200-400 ug; manganese – 300 mg; zinc – 30 mg |
| | **Biotin:** 16 mg daily |
| | **Onions and garlic** |
| | **Gymnema sylvestre:** 400 mg |

## PROSTATE ENLARGEMENT

**ALLOPATHIC**

**Surgery: TURP**
**Proscar**

**ALTERNATIVE**

**Diet:** low cholesterol, avoid beer and pesticides in food
**Amino acids:** glycine, alanine, glutamic acid – 360 mg daily
**Saw Palmetto:** 160 mg b.i.d.

## HEADACHE

**ALLOPATHIC**

**Acetylsalicylic acid (aspirin, etc.)**
Combinations: Fiorinal, etc.
**Acetaminophen (Tylenol, Anacin)**
Combinations: Fioricet
**Ergotamin**
**Sumatriptin**

**ALTERNATIVE**

**Diet:** avoid food allergies (milk, wheat, chocolate, cheese, and specifics; MSG (monosodium glutamate); nitrates: (artificially red-colored meats; alcohol (especially red wine)
**Avoid stress**
**Magnesium aspartate or citrate:** 350-500 mg. daily
**Feverfew:** as preventive – 25 mg b.i.d.; during attack – 1-2 gm
**Ginko biloba:** 80 mg. t.i.d.

## PEPTIC ULCER

| Allopathic | Alternative |
|---|---|
| **Antacids:** Calcium carbonate (Tums, etc.); Sodium bicarbonate: (Rolaids, Alka-Seltzer); Aluminum-magnesium hydroxide (Maalox, Mylanta, etc.) <br> **H-2 receptor antagonists** (Tagamet, Zantac, etc.) <br> **Bismuth** (Pepto-Bismol, etc.) | **Diet:** high fiber, avoid food allergies <br> **Life-style:** avoid stress, alcohol, smoking <br> **Vitamins/minerals:** A,C,E, zinc <br> **Avoid ASA and NSAID's** <br> **Deglycyrrhizinated licorice (DGL):** 2-4 380 mg tablets between or 20 min. before meals |

## REFERENCES

1. Stroehecker, J. (Exec. ed.) The Burton Goldberg Group. (1994). *Alternative medicine: The definitive guide.* Puyallup, WA: Future Medicine.
2. Guinness A. (Ed.) (1993). *Family guide to natural medicine.* Pleasantville, NY: Reader's Digest Association.
3. Gardner, M. (1995). Doug Henning and the giggling guru. *Skeptical Inquirer, 19* (3), 9-11/54.
4. Butler, K. (1992). *A consumer's guide to alternative medicine.* Buffalo, NY: Prometheus Books.
5. Skolnick, A. (1992). The Maharishi caper: JAMA hoodwinked (but just for a while). *Skeptical Inquirer, 16,* 254-259.
6. Huard, P., & Wong, M. (1968). *Chinese medicine.* London: World University Library.
7. Porkert, M. (1974). *The theoretical foundations of Chinese medicine – Systems of correspondence.* Cambridge, MA: MIT Press.

8. Brown, M.; Ulett, G.; & Stern, J. (1974). Acupuncture loci: Techniques for location. *Amer J Chin Med, 2* (1), 67-74.
9. Liu, K., et. al. (1975). The correspondence between some motor points and acupuncture loci. *Amer J Chin Med, 3,* 347-358.
10. Gunn, C. (1978). Motor points and motor lines. *Amer J Acup, 6,* 55-58.
11. Tollison, C., & Kriegel, M.(Eds.). (1989). *Rehabilitation of low back pain: A nonsurgical approach.* Baltimore: Williams & Wilkins.
12. Shekelle, P., & Brook, R. (1991). A community-based study of the use of chiropractic services. *Amer J Public Health, 81,* 439-442.
13. Shekelle, P., et. al. (1991). The appropriateness of spinal manipulation for low back pain. *RAND Publication Series, 1,* 29.
14. U.S. Public Health Service. (1994). *Clinical guide for treatment of low back pain.* Publication #95-0643. Rockville, MD.
15. Raso, J. (1995). Mystical medical alternativism. *Skeptical Inquirer, 19* (5), 33-37.
16. Fisher-Rizzi, S. *The complete aromatherapy handbook: Essential oils for radiant health.* New York: Sterling Press.
17. McCutcheon, L. (1995). Bach flower remedies: Time to stop smelling the flowers? *Skeptical Inquirer, 19* (4), 33-35.
18. Downing, G. (1972). *The massage book.* New York: Random House.
19. Barlow, W. (1991). *The Alexander technique.* New York: Alfred Knopf.
20. Feldenkreis, M., & Kimmey, M. (1992). *The potent self: A guide to spontaneity.* New York: Harper & Row.
21. Rolf, I. (1977). *Rolfing: The integration of human structures.* New York: Harper & Row.
22. Heller, J., & Henkin, W. (1991). *Bodywise.* Berkeley: Wingbow Press.
23. Trager, M., & Guadagno, C. (1987). *Trager mentastics: Movement as a way to agelessness.* New York: Station Hill Press.

24. Kunz, K., & Kunz, B. (1987). *Hand and foot reflexology: A self help guide.* New York: Simon & Schuster.
25. Gach, M. (1990). *Acupressure's potent points.* New York: Bantam Books.
26. Seidman, M. (1991). *Polarity therapy: The gentle art of hands-on healing.* Boulder, CO: Elan Press.
27. Krieger, D. (1993). *Your power to heal: Personal practice of therapeutic touch.* Santa Fe, NM: Bear & Company.
28. Upledger, J. (1992). *Your inner physician and you: CranioSacral therapy; SomatoEmotional release.* Berkeley, CA: North Atlantic Books.
29. Goodheart, G. (1989). *You'll be better: The story of applied kinesiology.* Geneva, OH: AK Printing.
30. Reich, W. (1949). *Character analysis.* New York: Noonday Press.

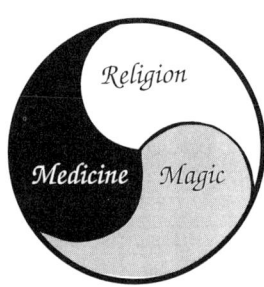

# VIII

# HERBOLOGY AND HOMEOPATHY
## THE PATH FROM HERBS TO DRUGS

HERBOLOGY, treatment by means of unrefined plants and other natural materials, had its origin with primitive tribes before the time of recorded history. From observing the effects of eating various plants by humans and animals, a folk knowledge gradually evolved that certain plants produced effects on the body. At times, some of these herbs would modify the course of an illness. Ultimately, these observations were recorded.

Perhaps the earliest record of the use of herbs was from clay tablets left by the Sumerians dating from 4000 B.C.E. In China, the *Pen Tsao* ("Great Herbs"), written about 3000 B.C.E., mentioned the medical use of 365 drugs, including *Papaver Somniferum*, the opium poppy, Ephedra for bronchial problems, and others. Impressive was the *Ebers Papyrus*, a 68-foot scroll found between the knees of an Egyptian mummy. It contained over 800 remedies, including not only plant extracts, but also animal substances, minerals, and descriptions of magical rites. Hippocrates (460-380 B.C.E.) preferred to let the patient recover naturally with diet, rest, and exercise, using laxatives, purgatives, and emetics sparingly. Roman historians recorded the use of plants for medicinal purposes. Perhaps the best known was Dioscorides, whose work, *De Materia Medica* (C.E. 77), describes the cultivation of some 600 plants with directions for their medicinal use. The Greek physician Galen (129-199 C.E.) had studied medicine at Pergamum, Smyrna, Corinth, and Alexandria. He was a surgeon to gladiators and the aristocracy. He contributed to knowledge of bodily functions and, as a druggist, based his formulations upon the Hippocratic belief in the four humors — blood, phlegm, and black and yellow bile. His complex formulae, known as "galenicals," were popular into the Middle Ages.

In Europe's Dark Ages (5th-11th Centuries), knowledge of herbology was recorded for the developing Arabic empire by scribes in Constantinople. Their great physicians, Rhazes (865-925) and Avicenna (930-1036), followed the doctrines of Hippocrates and Galen. In India, the herbal book of the Hindus, *Susruta,* appeared in the 5th Century.

During the Dark Ages in Europe, formulae for the use of drugs became mixed with ideas of superstition and magic. Bleeding by both bodily incisions and the use of leeches was popular. The latter gave name to herbal texts such as the famous *Leechbook of Bald* (900-950). Bald, like the witches of his time, believed in the existence of elves and goblins. The herbal brews of that time were not only directed at curing illness but also at protecting patients from the malbehaviour of supernatural creatures, e.g., for "a salve against the elfin race and nocturnal goblin visitors, take wormwood, lupin,...etc."

Around the 10th Century, monastic medicine came into being. Despite the fact that the Church Councils (1131-1212) prohibited monks from practicing medicine, the extensive libraries of the monasteries were repositories of herbal knowledge. Hospitals established at that time were primarily hospices which anointed the dying in preparation for death. Witches continued to practice medicine, and during the Inquisition, such witches — mostly women — were often put to death for their pagan healing practices. Encyclopedic works espoused the knowledge of the medical schools of Salerno and Montpelier. The *Liber de Proprietatibus Rerum* not only described medicinal plants, but also gave information on angels, demons, winged creatures, meteorology, cosmology, etc.

Paracelsus (born Theophrastus Bombastus von Hohenheim, near Zurich in 1493) has been called the "father of European pharmaceutical chemistry." His knowledge was gained from dealings with gypsies and midwives. As a youth, he worked in the mines of Tyrol, where he saw one metal used to purify another. He conceived the idea of using metals in this way to purify the human body. Later, as professor of medicine and city physician in Basle in 1527, he publicly burned the works of Galen and Avicenna.

Paracelsus was a follower of magic and alchemy, the latter being the belief in the transmutation of metals. The early Greeks and others thought that all substances were derived from one primitive matter. Mercury was a good candidate and was termed the *prima materia*. It had to be treated with sulfur to be freed from the four Aristotelian elements: earth, air, fire, and water. It was believed that if one could through "phlogistan," the spirit of fire, remove the red color from copper, one could produce silver. Paracelsus was rightly called the father of chemical science. Later the "al" was removed from the word alchemy and from these practices modern chemistry evolved. Today, "alchemy" is produced in physics laboratories by bombarding the atomic nucleus.

Although mainly famous for alchemy, Paracelsus used herbs combined with magical formulae. He believed that an herb resembling a body organ was specific for the treatment of that organ. He used the salts of heavy metals especially for the treatment of syphilis and also popularized the use of laudanum, the tincture of opium.

In 1568, William Turner published his *New Herbal*, dedicated to Queen Elizabeth I. It was the first scientific work to describe British flora, including over 200 native species with both botanical and herbal information.

After the voyages of Christopher Columbus, herbal texts contained descriptions of such newly discovered herbs as tobacco, sarsaparilla, and coca. By the 16th Century, many of the apothecaries had turned to alchemy, leaving to charlatans the prescribing of ointments, plasters and salves made of arsenic and mercury which were used for the treatment of syphilis. From the term "Quack Salver" for quicksilver or mercury came the term "quack" for those who used this method rather than the more popular use of herbs.

In 1617, the apothecaries residing in London who had been part of the Grocers' Company formed themselves into the Worshipful Society of the Art and Mystery of Apothecaries. The 17th Century saw a more ordered system for the prescription of drugs. In 1618, the first *London Pharmacopoeia* appeared, listing 1190 "simples," which were remedies consisting of a single drug. At this time, a genuine apothecary would have to serve a seven-year apprenticeship to practice as both a physician and a surgeon.

Belief in astrology was prominent, and prescriptions including metallic elements were associated with astrological signs, i.e., Saturn for lead, Mars for iron, Venus for copper, Hermes for tin, and Mercury for mercury. Such references even pertained to herbs. "Of hemlock," wrote Nicholas Culpepper (1616-1654), "Saturn claims dominion over this herb, yet I wonder why it may not be applied to the privities in a priapism, or continual standing of the yard, it being very beneficial to that disease." Culpepper supported the "doctrine of signatures," in which the shape of the plant and its resemblance to a body part determined its medicinal use. Thus the root of the orchid, which resembles the testes, was used for the treatment of testicular inflammation, "orchitis." Liver-shaped leaves were used for treatment of diseases of the liver, while red herbs, because of their color, were used for blood problems.

In 17th Century England, there was great preoccupation with digestive and bowel function. Hence, popular remedies were concerned with bimonthly purging. Such preoccupation was not new, however, as many centuries before, the *Ebers Papyrus* listed cathartics such as aloes, castor oil, senna, and rhubarb.

When the Pilgrims landed at Plymouth in 1630, they established herb gardens to replicate the herbal remedies which they had been using in England. They were surprised to find that the American Indians had their own herbs, such as cascara sagrada, goldenseal, and tobacco.

Publications at that time, both British and French, contained descriptions of gargles, pessaries, lotions, and liniments. In Europe, there were departments of pharmacy in the universities. The old ideas of Aristotle concerning the four elements were finally abandoned and chemical elements were defined as simple unitary substances. The 18th Century apothecaries were importers of raw materials which were converted into such preparations as tincture of Peruvian bark (for malaria) and cod liver oil (for rickets and rheumatism). William Withering's *An Account of the Foxglove and Some of its Medical Uses* (1785) was the first scientific account of the use of a folk remedy by a physician who listed a careful description of symptoms and doses.

The use of herbs came to the United States with the Pilgrims and other immigrants from Europe who brought with them the practice of growing herb gardens to meet the family's medical needs. Prominent among these were members of the United Society of Believers in Christ's Second

Coming, popularly known as "Shakers." They established the first herbal industry in the United States at Sabbath Lake, New Lebanon, New York, in 1799. In 1839, their catalog listed 160 species of medicinal herbs. They were the main suppliers of remedies to Samuel Thompson (1769-1843). This New Hampshire farmer-turned-healer claimed three million "Thompsonian" followers who formed "Friendly Botanical Societies" promoting the use of, primarily, lobelia, lady's slipper, bayberry bark, white water lily root, and butternut bark.

By the end of the 18th and the beginning of the 19th Century, there were major advances in the knowledge of chemistry, botany, and pharmacy. New techniques were developed that allowed the isolation of purer drugs from naturally occurring herbs. Mention was made of aconite, belladonna, cinchona, colchicum, hemlock, henbane, opium, and constituent alkaloids of these and other medicinal plants. Numerous small companies specializing in such plant extracts were set up in the late 19th Century. These were the forerunners of the modern pharmaceutical industry.

In Europe during the late 1800's, Pasteur and Koch were evolving the "germ theory," the basis for the development of therapeutics for infectious diseases. This was subsequently generalized as the "doctrine of specific etiology" to account for diseases other than those of infectious origin. Placebo controls in clinical trials performed the critical function of distinguishing medicine as a science and a profession. Hospital and laboratory-based experiments led to innovation and to patho-physiological explanation of disease. This provided medicine with technical superiority over other healing sects. It became clear that the core identity of pharmacological intervention was biochemical. Placebo medicine was identified and only later it became evident that the placebo effect of active drugs is masked by their more strictly physical effects (1).

It is difficult to determine how much of any drug's action is placebo and how much is specific. In China, we see a blending of ancient herbal wisdom and modern pharmaceutical knowledge. There it is common practice to use both Western types of medicine with substances whose use is supported only by ancient Chinese belief in herbal formulae. The latter are blended and packaged for the patient to take home and make into a broth that becomes the medication.

It is important to remember that the medicinal properties of plants vary not only with the time of year but also the time of day at which they are harvested. Flowers are fresher and more potent if picked in the morning before the sun has had time to dry them. Some plants are more potent if picked in the spring when the sap is flowing strongly. Roots may be better taken in the fall when they have progressed to a larger form. Such differences are not apparent when the dried herbs are purchased unless so stated on the labels. These differences in harvesting can account for major differences in the medicinal potency obtained from herbal medicines. There are also differences in potency according to how the products are prepared and whether dispensed in liquid or solid form. It is of interest that early remedies were mostly dry powders. Our word "drug" came from the Dutch word *drogge,* meaning "to dry."

**Human Physiology Dictates the Action of Drugs**

To understand the action of herbs and their purified derivatives or the synthetic facsimiles of modern drugs, one must look to the anatomy of the cells that make up the various systems of the body: heart and circulation, respiratory, digestive, reproductive, urinary, central nervous system, endocrine, structural (bone and muscle), and lymphatic. All of these are composed of cells. Each cell has a nucleus containing our hereditary material, the chromosomes, with their constituent genes. These are formed from molecules of deoxyribonucleic acid (DNA). The body is mostly made of water (up to 75%), which serves as the matrix containing the metals, sodium, potassium, and calcium, with some 20 or more trace chemicals and non-metallic substances including carbon, hydrogen, oxygen, nitrogen, sulphur, phosphorus, and chlorine. These are bound together with the DNA and RNA of the cell nucleus to form molecules of carbohydrates (sugars), lipids (fats), and proteins. Those molecules that are within the cells are protected by a cell membrane which consists of a layer of molecules formed into a latticework. At specific channels through this membrane, other molecules can pass, depending upon the action of the chemicals that guard such doors of entrance. Upon these cell membranes are certain molecular configurations known as "receptors." They are designed to receive or reject other molecules having a particular specific physical form. For example, a single drug molecule must have the physical shape to fit the receptor. Just as a key fits a lock, such medical molecules can "unlock" the specific channels of a cell and start a cascade of events that leads to changes in enzymes and body functions that then lead to healing. It is by this method that different body systems communicate with each other.

Body energy, the "mysterious life forces" about which the ancients pondered, and upon which they formed their basic philosophical concepts of medical systems, is now recognized (a) as the action of molecules such as hormones and enzymes that travel through the body, and (b) of the central nervous system. Function of the nervous system is dependent upon a complex set of events that occurs at the synaptic junction, a cleft that separates one nerve cell from another. The pre-synaptic (sending) neuron releases, through its cellular membrane, substances which act upon the surface of the post-synaptic (receiving) neuron. Ultimately, this opens channels in the long nerve cell process (axon) that permits the passage of sodium ions into the interior, potassium-rich central process of the axon. This alteration permits a change in the surface charge of the axon from a positive to a negative electrical potential and sends an electrical message along the axon to activate muscles or organ functions.

Some of these molecular keys serve to open channels, while others close channels. Some are activators increasing a body function, while some serve to slow or even stop body processes. Some speed up enzymatic actions, others slow them down. Observations of the results of such physiological activities were the basis of primitive beliefs in "life force" or "body energy."

It is within this biochemical test tube, the body, that the molecules of the treating substance must act. To the ancient herbologists, this was a confusing mystery, explained only in terms of the philosophical concepts of that era. Thanks to modern pharmacology and biochemistry, our understanding of these processes has become increasingly clear. Each of the thousands of plant remedies made up of complex molecular structure, representing molecules of many varieties, may have within it a single type of active molecule that can act upon a specific type of cell receptor. Hence, the multi-ingredient formulae of many ancient herbal preparations must be viewed with caution.

It is only within this century that pharmacologists have been able to use the advances of biochemistry and physiology to determine the site and manner of action of purified drugs. Prior to this time, herbologists were only guessing at what might be going on in the body. They had only the verbal reports and anecdotes of patients, their families, and the observations of the relatively unskilled and untrained health providers of that pre-scientific era. Some of these made remarkably good guesses that led to separating out the herbs that appeared to have a definite action. Following such leads, about 25% of today's modern drugs have been developed by the extraction and purification of crude plant materials. This process has removed from the complicated organic matter of the plant those materials that are noncontributing to the healing action or that are toxic in nature.

Most drugs can be toxic or even lethal if the dose is not carefully regulated. In the United States, the Federal Drug Administration (FDA) has established stringent testing procedures which each new drug must undergo prior to its approval for prescription use. Drugs that are approved have been rigorously tested so that impurities are removed, safe dosing schedules have been established, and whatever side effects may occur are limited and known to the prescribing physician. Schwartz (2) has pointed out that of 5,000 compounds chemically tested, only 500 make it to the testing stage. Of these, 250 are tested in animals and five make it to human trials. Of these, one receives FDA approval. This process takes several years and can cost over 200 million dollars.

Patients often complain that drugs that have already been studied in foreign countries are held up for long delays before they can be used in the United States. It should be pointed out, however, that even the safest-appearing drugs may have long-term side effects. An example is Thalidomide, introduced from Europe into the United States with devastating results of fetal anomalies. If we were to accept lower standards, we would at the same time be accepting a higher risk of morbidity and mortality. When persons seek to obtain from foreign countries drugs that are not yet licensed in the United States, they are taking the risk of experiencing possible serious consequences. The extra safety measures mandated by the FDA result in higher costs in the manufacture of drugs. These extra costs, incurred for the safety of the consumer, account for a higher price of such medication.

Drugs are protected by patent for 17 years, after which they are released for manufacture by companies that did not develop the drug. This patent protection is offered in order for the pharmaceutical corporation that developed the new drug to have the opportunity to regain the great development cost it has experienced. Also, as a private industry, it is entitled to a reasonable profit. When this patent time expires, other companies can manufacture and sell this drug. As these other corporations did not incur the heavy developmental costs, they can sell such "generic" drugs at a lower price. In most cases, these drugs are chemically identical to the original non-generic drug. In a few instances, differences in the manufacturing process may result in the generic drug having a lesser potency or some side effects not seen with the original drug.

As individuals differ greatly in their physiology and biochemistry, they may also differ in the amount of medicine they require for a given illness and their susceptibility to side effects. Thus, the administration of drugs is not a standard procedure but rather it is the essence or "art" of medicine in which the physician seeks to match the patients' needs in selecting from the many drugs available. For any illness there may be several drugs that can have the same desired effect. Some may be more likely than others to cure, but may also be more likely to produce side effects. Here, the physician must make a decision regarding the health benefit compared to the risk of side effects. Because all drugs have multiple side effects, patients frequently complain about the "drugging" of allopathic medicine. This may be one factor that leads them to risk the more exotic, less understood, and magical offerings of herbal medicine, whose weak formulations may avoid toxic reactions, but at the same time provide questionable medicinal action.

Despite glowing promotions and statements to the contrary by some advocates, natural plants can produce as many side effects as synthetic drugs. In fact, since the latter have been carefully screened and tested, they would appear to be safer than so called "natural" herbs that are presently classified as foods and therefore have escaped the rigor of testing for toxicity and dose specificity. Also, the plants themselves, unlike the extracted and purified drugs obtained from them, are composed of many constituent substances. Herb formulations often contain not one, but a number of plants. Selecting at random from a catalog of herb remedies, for example, one encounters descriptions such as:

> ...indicated for persons with headaches, dizziness, flank pain, and tiredness...for gynecological problems such as irregular and painful menses and breast distention ...indispensable formula for

regulating the flow of women's blood...can be used for digestive problems...including such symptoms as loose stools, gas, distention, bloating, and chronic stomach ache.

The above advertised concoction is made up of the following constituents: Hare's Ear root, Tang Kuei root, Peony root, Atractylodes, Tuckahoe, Peppermint, Licorice root, Tree Peony root bark, Gardenia fruit, Szechuan Lovage root, Gastrodia rhizome, Nut Grass rhizome, and Ginger rhizome.

Lest it appear that the above is atypical, one could have selected any from among the multitude of such recommended herbal formulas listed in the catalogs of herbal pharmaceutical companies. In this, as in others, it is important to note the great number of plants included in the formula. Each one of these plants includes various fibers and miscellaneous constituents of unknown value. Questionable also is the "cure-all" nature of this "shotgun" formula, acting, as it claims, upon the digestive, nervous, and reproductive systems, and recommended as well for a variety of painful conditions. Taking such an herbal product without first obtaining a proper diagnosis of one's illness could be most unwise. Symptoms so treated could represent manifestations of cancer or other conditions requiring immediate surgical attention or specific medication.

The above suggests why one must be particularly wary of the so-called "green wave" of interest in herbology that is increasing in the United States today. Such turning away from allopathic medicine may be prompted by the patient with a chronic illness that has not responded to the administration of some specific medicine. Or possibly, there may be discontent from a lack of warmth and adequate communication by a busy physician. Perhaps the patient has experienced some distressing side effects from a prescribed drug or is lured by the fantastic claims of New Age ads. The above situations are remedied by patience and discussion, but are not good reasons to forsake treatment by modern medicines that have been developed through hard-won scientific knowledge resulting in meaningful diagnostic and prescribing techniques.

Some herbalists or homeopathic physicians are M.D.'s and D.O.'s with full knowledge of and skills in modern allopathic medicine. They are fully capable of using the best diagnostic methods and, if they wish an alternative to herbs, are equipped to use more appropriate specific drugs and scientific methods. Because the prescription and use of herbal preparations are not regulated in the U.S. by the Federal Drug Administration, they fall under the classification of foodstuffs. Thus, herbal remedies may be prescribed by persons having no medical knowledge. It is evident that the administration of herbal preparations can thus be fraught with danger.

Apart from inappropriate use which may prolong or aggravate symptoms, the herbs themselves could contain toxic materials, have numerous side effects, and be administered in minuscule, ineffective doses in order to minimize toxicity. Such doses then may not be effective beyond the placebo actions that have sustained their use through the Dark Ages.

On the plus side, however, the hundreds of herbs that have been studied and the thousands more awaiting harvest and study from forests around the world contain chemicals that form the basis for the modern pharmaceutical industry. Table III lists a few of the herbs whose active principles through scientific methods have resulted in the development of prescription drugs. In many cases, a knowledge of the molecular structure of active derivatives has permitted not only the development of similar but also more effective substances. Modern pharmaceutical manufacturing processes have produced medicines more cheaply and in volumes that would have been impossible through agricultural methods.

While naturopaths, homeopaths, and others rail against the high cost of prescription drugs and the large profits of major pharmaceutical corporations, they remain silent about the profits, abuses, and false claims made by manufacturers of the herbal preparations they recommend (in which, incidentally, they may have a proprietary interest). There is no doubt that prescription drugs are costly and certainly, in part, because of the millions of dollars that must be spent to protectively determine toxicity and dosage before putting a drug on the market. Such expenses, with the 13% average profit margin, add to the high cost of medical care in Western countries. Manufacturers of herbal preparations sold as "foods" do not have these large pre-market costs and thus the price seems less by comparison with prescription drugs. However, the profit margins can be even greater. As such herbal products become increasingly popular, they, too, will add greatly to the cost of medical care.

Having been for decades "detailed" by the salespersons of major pharmaceutical concerns, I can only say that I am impressed by not only the knowledge they have of their own products, but also an understanding of the biochemical and physiological actions that they have gained from corporate training seminars. The advertisements for their products are often backed by statistics complete with references from comparative double-blind studies.

By comparison, the sales promotions of herbal remedies leave much to be desired. I am seldom visited by herbal sales representatives with whom I could discuss the relative merits of their preparations. Rather, I am bombarded by catalogs filled with the most extravagant claims. Rarely indicated are the results of controlled or double-blind studies of herbs published by reputable researchers in peer-reviewed journals. No rationale is presented for dosing schedules, and no scientific studies of drug action or detailed discussion of possible side effects. All too often, the remedies are listed by some fanciful name such as "The Woman's Tonic," or "Masculinity Regained," thus implying vague but marvelous healing properties, but with no indication as to which of the many ingredients in the compound may be responsible for what action.

An important factor in formulating a standard basis for pharmaceutical practice was the establishment by the AMA of its Council on Pharmacy and Chemistry, which investigated all compounds submitted by various companies for the use of physicians. This was a significant attempt to overcome the abuses that accompanied the unregulated sale of nostrums, compounds of mixed effective and non-effective substances which characterized medicine in the late 19th and early 20th Centuries (3). In Europe, herbs are widely used under the term "phytotherapy" or "botanical medicine." In Germany, herbology is taught in all medical schools, and physicians must pass an examination in the use of herbs in order to obtain their license to practice medicine. The World Health Organization estimates that 80% of the world's population is dependent upon its indigenous traditional medicine, the largest element of which is the use of herbal substances (4).

Table IV lists some of the most popular and widely used natural remedies. These are readily obtainable in pharmacies in Europe and other parts of the world. Local terms for herbs vary widely and it is best to seek them by their botanical names. Although some herbs are beginning to become available in drug stores of the U.S., natural food stores are still the main source of supply.

Herbal remedies vary widely in their potency, depending upon the part of the plant used, its method of growth, and the time of harvesting. The term "Certified Organically Grown" means that one of the several third-party certifying agencies has assured that the product has been grown without the use of synthetic pesticides, herbicides, or chemical fertilizers. Methods of preparation, too, are important. Herbs may be purchased in their raw form as bark, roots, flowers, or seeds. They may be ground or powdered. Herb powders in capsules have some delay in absorption, but do not contain the added substances necessary to form pills. Number 0 capsule contains about 10 grains of the herb, number 00 about 15 grains.

Infusions and teas are made by adding boiling water to the powdered herb. Decoctions are made by seeping and simmering. Tinctures are very concentrated extracts of the herb in liquid form. They are prepared by maceration, percolation, or extraction with alcohol. Later, the alcohol may be distilled off. As heat can destroy some of the herb's potency, it may be preferable to leave the small amount of alcohol that remains. Syrups and salves are made with organic additives such as malt syrup and honey, maple syrup, cocoa fat, or vegetable oil. Less commonly used today are poultices in which the herb in paste form is placed on a cloth bandaged against the skin to promote absorption.

Shelf life, too, is important with powders, capsules, and tea bags retaining potency for up to six months, tablets and dried leaves up to a year, dried roots three years, and liquid extracts 10-20 years.

## Modern Pharmaceuticals

The last half-century has seen tremendous advances in medical science, including the important development of designer drugs, which have produced cures of diseases that have seemed almost miraculous. In the field of psychiatry, for example, prior to the 1930's, patients with serious depression and manic depressive illness were simply locked up, placed in restraints, and subjected to a variety of harsh and worthless treatment methods. The length of hospital stay was measured in months, recoveries were not assured, and suicide was common. With the advent of electroshock therapy, hospital time was reduced and recoveries were dramatic. However, vertebral fractures were a common complication. The introduction of the South American arrow poison, curare, softened the convulsions that were a part of such treatments, but some fractures still occurred. Curare was later replaced by better synthetics such as anectine, which virtually eliminated fractures. In the 1960's, a series of designer anti-depressants, the tri-cyclics, and later, specific serotonin reuptake inhibitors (SSRI's) and others were introduced. Now, 90% of depressed patients are quickly relieved of the symptoms of their depression by pharmaceutical intervention. With careful monitoring and matching the drug to the patient, distressing side effects are rare.

Another mental illness, schizophrenia, affects one in a hundred persons. Until the 1950's, no good treatment existed for most of these patients who spent a large part of their lives sequestered in mental hospitals. The development of synthetic drugs, the psycholeptics, produced a dramatic change in the lives of these patients. First came chlorpromazine, and then later a host of others with good anti-psychotic actions and differing side effects. Many of these patients are now able to leave the hospital and return to the community. For some chronic patients, the development of distressing repetitive motor movements in the form of Parkinsonian symptoms, and later, the onset of Tardive Dyskinesia, has limited the usefulness of these drugs. Some newer agents — like clozapine and risperidone, for example — have eliminated this problem for another 25% of patients.

Similar stories can be told in almost every branch of medicine. There are dozens of new designer cardiac drugs with an outstanding record of controlling high blood pressure and preventing heart disease. Successes have been obtained with new drugs for peptic ulcer, pain, and arthritis. Many of these owe their existence to early derivatives from natural plants. Once the essential ingredient of the herbal remedy was discovered, it led to successive purifications and the design of more effective synthetic compounds. Today, modern pharmaceutical companies are searching the rain forests for new herbs to explore in their laboratories. In China, there is an ongoing review of the centuries-old herbal remedies, with refining and experimentation leading to the discovery of the essence of ancient formulae. Purification and testing are leading to the development of new "scientific" medications.

The undisciplined use of ancient formulae, mixtures of strange and too-often untested plants with unknown composition, is in reality a trip back to the Dark Ages. Rather, we should look upon herbs as the forerunners of modern medicines. Modern pharmacology owes its lifesaving scientific methods to the centuries-old use of herbal remedies.

It is, of course, up to the patient to either seek the best that modern scientific medicine has produced or risk the possibility of turning back the clock to the days of superstition and folk medicine with drugs parlayed under such titles as "holistic" or "natural."

Table IV lists some of the more widely used herbal preparations. Although it is estimated that there are over 250,000 plants, only about 5,000 of these have been studied for possible use in medical practice. The Chinese pharmacopeia alone lists some 1,600 separate natural items used in the practice of Traditional Chinese Medicine. The 45 preparations listed here were selected as the ones most frequently used and favorably supported by reason of long usage, safety, and some acceptable documentation of their usefulness by writers of texts on herbology. They should be used with caution, as they have not been approved by the FDA's rigorous program of testing for toxicity.

Because herbal preparations are only now coming again to the attention of allopathic physicians, reports are beginning to appear in medical journals about not only their potential therapeutic value, but also of possible hazards associated with their use. Drugs and herbs are basically toxic to human tissues; it is only in dilute form that some of them have the useful side effects that have led to their therapeutic use. The screening process is rigorous. Just because something is called "natural" does not mean that it is benign. Recently warnings have been published about some commonly used herbal preparations. Among these are *germander, chaparral leaf,* and *comfrey.* A number of traditional remedies including clam shell powder *(Hai Ge Fen)* from China, *azarcon* or *greta* (Hispanic), *paylooah* (Southeast Asian), *surma* (Indian), and others have been sources of lead poisoning in children. Similarly, hepatoxicity has been found with some Chinese topical preparations. There are many Chinese and Indian herbal clinics in England. Here, problems arise from poor control of imports, difficulty in identifying herbal products, addition to herbals of potent steroids, and other contaminant factors.

In one example of ambiguity, Kleinjen (5) reports that

> ...evening primrose oil has not been proved efficacious in rigorous clinical trials...nevertheless, evening primrose oil is an interesting substance, and for some indications it is a promising treatment — especially for diabetic neuropathy and atopic dermatitis, but as for rheumatoid arthritis and the premenstrual syndrome, further rigorous trials of both evening primrose oil and gamma linolenic acid are warranted.

**Homeopathy**

Hippocrates, the Greek "father of Western medicine" who lived in the 5th Century B.C.E., was the first to record in his writings the homeopathic principle that "like cures like." In 1811, Samuel Hahnemann, a physician in Leipzig, published a detailed system of healing based on this principle of *similia similibus curentur*. Hahnemann was disillusioned with the way medicine was being practiced. He travelled and taught Greek, Hebrew, and Arabian, and thus became familiar with the works of the 16th Century Paracelsus, who believed strongly in magical cures and was a supporter of the belief in "similars," in which the shape of the plant indicated its use for the body organ it most resembled.

An Englishman returning from Peru introduced Hahnemann to the bark of the cinchona tree, which had cured him of malaria. Hahnemann chewed some of the bark and promptly had symptoms of fever, palpitations, flushing, and thirst, symptoms similar, he thought, to those of the disease malaria. From this, he developed the idea that what cures a sick person will also produce the same symptoms of illness in a healthy person. Using this principle, he tested hundreds of substances on healthy volunteers, observing any deviations from the normal that were produced. He matched the symptoms of his patients to the symptoms produced by the substances he had tested. These observations he called "provings." In this way, during his lifetime he defined some 4,000 homeopathic remedies.

Homeopathy made its first impact upon American and European medicine during the Asiatic cholera epidemic of 1832. At this time, prior to the development of any antibiotics, it was observed that the patients of homeopaths had a far higher rate of recovery than those treated by the harsh methods used by other healers. Homeopathy grew during the late

19th and early 20th Centuries. The first homeopathic college opened in Philadelphia in 1836. The American Institute of Homeopathy, formed in 1844, was the first national medical organization in the United States. By the end of the century, there were 15,000 practicing homeopaths and 22 homeopathic schools in the country.

In the early years of the 20th Century, the scientific approach to medicine was as yet new, and belief in unproven medical procedures was widespread. John D. Rockefeller, for example, was sympathetic to homeopathy, and it was only through the persuasion of his son and staff that he was convinced that homeopathy was based on "pre-conceived notions," while allopathic medicine was "devoid of dogma of any kind." Thus, the Rockefeller Institute for Medical Research was founded (6).

At that time, there was a struggle for dominance between homeopathy and allopathic medicine. With the development of modern pharmaceutical techniques, the introduction of antibiotics, and advances in diagnostic and surgical procedures, the ancient practice of homeopathy gradually declined. The last school of homeopathic medicine, Hahnemann Medical School in Philadelphia, changed its full curriculum to allopathic medicine in the 1930's. In the last two decades, however, with the increasing interest in alternative medicine, the teaching of homeopathy is again on the rise.

Major principals of homeopathic theory are: *1)* the "Law of Similars"; *2)* provings; *3)* trituration and succussion; *4)* potentization or the "Law of Infinitesimals"; and *5)* "miasma."

Under the **law of similars**, the physician must seek the remedy whose symptomatology is precisely similar to that of the patient's illness. Thus, it is essential that in diagnosing the illness of a patient, the physician seeks to delineate the fine and subtle differences that characterize the individual patient's illness. The homeopathic physician aims to treat "the whole" patient and spends a long time taking a history that searches out unique aspects of the patient's physical being, emotions, likes, dislikes, and behavior, as well as any peculiar symptoms that are manifest. The remedy that matches most precisely the unique personality and symptoms of the patient is selected from the several thousand remedies available.

Homeopaths like to point out that this "law of similars" resembles the practice of vaccination used in allopathic medicine. There are, however, major differences. Vaccines are strong, not weak. They are not just similar, but are made from the actual organism that causes the illness. Also, they are given not to treat an illness that is present but rather to prevent later occurrence of the disease for which the patient has been vaccinated.

Each of the homeopathic remedies has undergone extensive "**provings**," in which the drug has been tested by administration to healthy volunteers who recorded every mental, emotional, and physical effect that occurred. These symptoms are then attributed to the specific drug to be matched to the symptoms of any patient with an illness that shows those symptoms. The drug must not only match the symptoms of the illness but also the personal characteristics of the patient.

The healing magic of the homeopathic medication also depends upon the manner in which the remedy is prepared. Non-soluble preparations are crushed and diluted with lactose (**trituration**). Soluble preparations are diluted with alcohol or water. Vigorous shaking (**succussion**) is thought to increase potency.

A major unproven guiding principle of homeopathy is that the smaller the dose, the greater the potency of the medicine (**potentization**). In this, the solution of the drug is subjected to serial dilutions up to the tenth power, or a dilution to 1/1000 of the original solution. At this point, according to Avagdro's law, probably not one molecule of the original substance remains. Homeopaths believe, however, that somehow the initial substance has left its imprint on the molecules of water or alcohol so that they can "resonate" with the symptoms in the patient's body. As Butler (7) points out, "...if homeopathy were true, there could be no chemistry as we know it because there would be no pure substances—every substance would imprint its vibes forever on everything it ever came in contact with."

The concept of **miasma** refers to the belief that persons can inherit the tendency to acquire diseases that have been experienced by their parents. Thus, for example, if a relative had gonorrhea, one might develop symptoms that are known to occur with that illness. This aberrant belief in acquired diseases was probably derived from the observation that certain tendencies for some diseases do run in families, e.g., cancer, diabetes, hypertension, etc. These are, however, genetically inherited, not acquired tendencies. Homeopathy distinguishes five miasmas: psychotic, tuberculinic, psoric, syphilitic, and canceric.

Perhaps the greatest asset of the homeopathic physician is the doctor/patient relationship that develops from the prolonged history-taking. A common complaint from patients of allopathic physicians is that "my doctor does not listen to my complaints." Also, homeopaths, following the lead of Hahnemann, are holistic in their treatment approach, trusting in the body's own healing powers assisted by exercise, fresh air, diet, and vitamins.

Many homeopathic remedies are made from poisonous substances and are given for illness produced by those substances, e.g., lead for lead poisoning, mercury for mercuric poisoning. Because the remedies are so greatly diluted, little harm seems to result. Homeopaths see symptoms as a positive sign of the body trying to defend itself against the disease. They therefore believe that an illness may get worse before getting better. They differ from orthodox physicians, whom they claim suppress diseases with strong medicine, thus interfering with the body's natural healing processes. In this matter, the danger of such homeopathic thinking lies in a failure to treat serious illness with known curative agents, thus allowing a disease to progress to a stage in which it may become potentially fatal.

## Naturopathy

Although homeopathy as a single technique has been added to the practice of many chiropractors and acupuncturists, it is a mainstay of naturopathy. The underlying theme of naturopaths, like that of homeopaths, is that all disease is a result of the failure of natural body defense mechanisms. Therefore, treatment by naturopaths is designed to restore the body's own ability to fight the disease rather than use harsher methods to stifle the symptoms. Often, treatment is aimed at increasing rather than decreasing the symptoms of illness that are seen as the body's inadequate attempts to fight the disease.

Naturopaths claim to have included in their practice the healing wisdom of such ancient cultures as Greece (Hippocratic), India (Ayurveda), China (Traditional Chinese Medicine), and Native America. From this background, they have evolved six major principles (4):

1. **The healing power of nature:** To facilitate the patient's ability to heal using natural, non-toxic therapies.

**2. Treat the cause rather than the effect:** Symptoms are viewed as the body's attempt to heal itself. The cause of the illness is sought in physical, mental/emotional, and spiritual areas.

**3. First, do no harm:** Employ only safe, natural remedies.

**4. Treat the whole person:** Patient is viewed as a complex interaction of emotional, physical, spiritual, social, and other factors. Treatment includes attention to all of these.

**5. The physician is a teacher:** Educate, motivate, and empower the patients to assume personal responsibility for their own health by adopting healthy attitudes, life-styles, and diets.

**6. Prevention is the best cure:** Teach each patient a life-style that is healthy.

Naturopaths see themselves as a type of general practitioner or family physician who specializes in holistic medicine. Their degree, N.D., Doctor of Naturopathic Medicine, is granted by one of the four new U.S. schools of naturopathic medicine (Seattle, WA, Portland, OR, Concord, NH, and Scottsdale, AZ). The four-year curriculum consists of training in: homeopathy; clinical nutrition; botanical medicine; acupuncture; physical medicine, including hydrotherapy, physiotherapy, and manipulative techniques; psychological counseling; and minor surgery. Seven states (Alaska, Arizona, Connecticut, Hawaii, Montana, Oregon, and Washington) and the District of Columbia have specific licenses for Naturopaths. They may also practice in other states that have right-to-practice laws. They are tolerated in some other states.

Licensure of Naturopaths probably occurs because legislators are unaware that their practice includes techniques having no scientific basis. In pursuing licensure, naturopaths, like other holistic healers, use vague and unscientific phrases to explain what they do. For example, Hawaiian law describes naturopathy as

> ...the practice of natural medicine, natural therapeutics, and natural procedures, for the purpose of removing toxic conditions from the body and improving the quality, quantity, harmony, balance, and flow of the vital fluids, vital tissues, and vital energy; and the practice of diagnosing, treating, and caring for patients using a system of practice that bases its treatment of physiological functions and abnormal conditions on natural laws governing the human body.

Such a statement vaguely defines almost any practice of healing.

Who can be against that which is "natural" when the opposite of that term is "unnatural"? In his *Consumers Guide to Alternative Medicine*, Kurt Butler (7) states, "Naturopathy is a pseudoscientific healing cult and a hazard to the public's health. It has a symbiotic and unethical relationship with the health food and natural therapeutics industry, the makers and wholesalers of the snake oils they use."

It is not that some of the techniques used by naturopaths are in themselves without value. Here, as elsewhere in the field of Alternative Medicine, however, the practitioner should be able to properly diagnose those conditions that are serious and known to respond well to recognized orthodox scientific methods. Perhaps the four years of study would be better done in an allopathic school of medicine with later specialization in those techniques which could, where appropriate, be used adjunctively.

Apart from the use of techniques of questionable scientific validity, one must recognize that the basic principles of naturopathy represent an ideal to which all practitioners of the healing arts should subscribe. These are: an emphasis on looking at the whole person, using methods that produce as little harm as possible; and educating the patient toward a more healthful life-style. This would be therapeutic and preventive medicine at its best.

## REFERENCES

1. Sullivan, M. (1993). Placebo controls and epistemic control in orthodox medicine. *J Med and Phil, 18*, 213-231.
2. Schwartz, A. (1992, September). 5,000 tries = one new drug. *US Pharm, 8*, 9.
3. Burrow, J. (1977). *Organized medicine in the bygone era: The trend toward monopoly*. Baltimore: John's Hopkins University Press.
4. The Burton Goldberg Group. Strohecker, J. (Ex.ed.). (1994). *Alternative medicine: The definitive guide*. Puyallup, WA: Future Medicine Publishing.
5. Kleinjen, J. (1994). Evening primrose oil: Currently used in many conditions with little justification. *Brit Med J, 309*, 824-825.
6. Brown, R. (1980). *Rockefeller medicine men*. Berkeley, CA: University of California Press.

7. Butler, K. (1992). *A consumer's guide to "alternative medicine."* Buffalo, NY: Prometheus Books.

## TABLE III

| PRIMITIVE DRUG | MODERN DERIVATIVE |
| --- | --- |
| Chincona bark | Quinine |
| Foxglove | Digitalis |
| Willow bark | Salicylates |
| Woody nightshade | Cancer research drugs |
| Sheep sorrel | Oxalic acid |
| Mold preparations | Penicillin |
| Coca leaves | Cocaine |
| Buckthorn bark | Cascara |
| Opium poppy | Morphine |
| Evergreen leaves (Ephedra) | Ephedrine |
| Hecogenin agave | Cortisone |
| Diosgenin | Prednisone |
| Ergot | Ergonovine, methysergide |
| Corynanthe yohimbe | Yohimbine |
| Rauwolfia | Reserpine |
| Moldy clover | Dicoumarol |
| Ammi visnaga | Sodium cromoglycate |
| Cephaelis acuminata | Ipecac, emetine |
| Colchicum autumnale | Colchine |
| Cantharanthus roseus | Vincristine |
| Trichoderma inflatum | Cyclosporin |
| Taxus baccata | Taxol |

# TABLE IV

## SOME WIDELY USED NATURAL REMEDIES *

**ALOE VERA** *(Aloe barbidensis)* Its clear sticky gel is applied directly over wounds or burns. Said to help regenerate new tissue and aid healing. Beware skin irritation in sensitive persons. Used internally for ulcer. Dried juice as a cathartic.

**ANISE** *(Pimpinella anisum)* A flavoring, digestive aid for colic, and for coughs as a syrup or lozenge.

**BASIL** *(Ocimum basilicum)* As a carminative to relieve stomach cramps and gas.

**CASCARA SAGRADA** *(Rhamnus purshiana)* Bark from the tree found in the Northwest. Dried for one year; is used as an ingredient in laxatives.

**CATNIP** *(Napeta cateria)* As a somnolent tea. A member of the mint family, aids digestion.

**CAYENNE** *(Capsicum annum)* Rubificient, increases sweating. Aids digestion. Used externally as a poultice for painful joints. Acts by interfering with peripheral pain conduction.

**CHAMOMILE** *(Matricaria chamomillia)* Carminative, anti-spasmodic and sleep aid. Anti-inflammatory when applied to the skin. Beware in persons with ragweed allergies.

**CINNAMON** *(Cinnamomum zeylanicum)* Appetite stimulant and carminative, relieves gas and stomach upset, nausea, and vomiting. Also for diarrhea.

**CRANBERRY** *(Vaccinium macrocarpon)* Prevention of urinary infections.

**ECHINACEA** *(Echinacea angustifolia)* Ancient American Indian remedy. Anti-infective and immuno-stimulant. For treatment and prevention of the common cold. Externally for wound healing.

*continued*

**EUCALYPTUS** *(Eucalyptus globulus)* To clear mucus and assist with respiratory problems. As a vapor, rub, or lozenge.

**EVENING PRIMROSE** *(Oenothera biennis)* Long touted as a "cure-all." Probably useful for atopic asthma and excema, migraine, and pre-menstrual tension.

**FENNEL** *(Foeniculum vulgare)* Anti-spasmodic for flatulence and to aid digestion.

**FEVERFEW** *(Tanacetum parthenium)* Use the leaves fresh or frozen or herbal powder. Prevention of migraine headaches.

**GARLIC** *(Allium sativum)* Best used fresh. Becomes active when cut or crushed. Treatment of atherosclerosis and high blood pressure. Boosts immune function. An effective anti-microbial against bacteria, viruses, worms, and fungi. Effective against *Candida albicans*. Helps with blood clotting. Good for gastro-intestinal disorders.

**GINGER** *(Zingiber officinale)* For nausea and motion sickness. Aids digestion, stimulates salivation and gastric secretions, and reduces gas and intestinal spasms. Increases the effectiveness of other medicines. Migraine relief.

**GINKGO** *(Ginko biloba)* Comes from the oldest species of tree in the world. Increases peripheral and brain circulation. Vascular diseases, pulmonary diseases, tinnitus, and short-term memory loss.

**GINSENG** Oriental *(Panex ginseng),* American *(Panex quinquefolius).* Siberian ginseng *(Eleutherococcus senticosus)* also known as Eulethro. Pseudo-ginseng *(Paneax pseudoginseng)*. The word *Panex is* derived from the Greek *panacea* meaning cure-all. An adaptogen or tonic useful for combating the effects of stress. Claims to overcome fatigue. Highly praised in the Orient for numerous maladies. If taken in excess, can prove toxic.

*continued*

**GOLDENSEAL** *(Hydrastis canadensis)* A tonic remedy that stimulates the immune system. Contains berberine and other alkaloids that are antimicrobial. Not as powerful as modern antibiotics but has been shown effective against *Staphylococcus, Streptococcus, Candida albicans,* and *Giardia lambila.* Colds, flu and genito-urinary infections. Mouthwash for cracked lips and canker sores.

**HAWTHORN** *(Crataegus oxycantha)* Dilates blood vessels and lowers blood pressure. Strengthens heart. Mild sedative.

**HOPS** *(Humulus lupulus)* Contains an alcohol used in brewing beer. Useful sedative and anti-anxiety agent. Dried hops are used as a pillow-aid in sleeping. Anti-spasmodic to ease diarrhea and intestinal cramps. Fresh plant can cause allergy.

**HYSSOP** *(Hyssopus officinalis)* A carminative member of the mint family. Expectorant for coughs and colds. Aids digestion of fats.

**LICORICE** *(Glycyrrhiza glabra)* Expectorant, demulcent, good for coughs and colds. Anti-inflammatory action, recommended for treatment of peptic ulcer. Increases sodium retention and can raise blood pressure.

**MA HUANG** *(Ephedra sinica)* Anti-asthmatic. Allergy and flu symptoms. Caution advised, as is a central nervous system stimulant.

**MILK THISTLE** *(Silybum marianum)* Viral hepatitis. Liver protectant.

**MYRRH** *(Commiphora molmol)* Astringent and antiseptic useful for cleansing wounds and bedsores. As a mouthwash for sore throats and gingivitis.

**NETTLE** *(Urtica dioica)* Diuretic.

**PARSLEY** *(Petroselinum crispum)* Digestive aid, diuretic, emmenagogue. Sweetens breath.

*continued*

**PASSION FLOWER** *(Pasiflora incarnata)* For insomnia. Sedative, calmative.

**PEPPERMINT** *(Mentha piperita)* For indigestion, colic and gas. Appetite stimulant.

**PSYLLIUM** *(Plantago ovata)* A soothing bulk-producing laxative. Useful for constipation and irritable bowel syndrome.

**ROSE HIPS** *(Rosa canina)* Anti-scorobutic.

**ROSEMARY** *(Rosmarinus officinalis)* Culinary herb. Mild laxative and diuretic. Mild painkiller for headaches and stomach pain. Contains antibacterial agent (rosmaricine), which stimulates smooth muscles.

**SAGE** *(Salvia officinalis)* As an astringent gargle for tonsillitis, bleeding gums, and inflammatory conditions of mouth and throat. Can decrease perspiration, but beware, as large dosage taken internally can cause convulsions.

**SAW PALMETTO** *(Serenoa repens)* Prostatic enlargment, urinary obstruction, and male urinary problems.

**SENNA** *(Cassia angustifolia)* A stimulant laxative. Avoid in pregnancy.

**SLIPPERY ELM** *(Ulmus fulva)* A salve for skin injuries, burns, and chapped lips. Lozenge for sore throats and cough.

**ST. JOHN'S WORT** *(Hypericum perforatum)* Sedative properties. Anti-anxiety, anti-depressant. Anti-inflammatory under investigation as anti-viral compound. Beware photosensitivity reaction.

**THYME** *( Thymus vulgaris)* A versatile healing seasoning. Decreases gastric discomfort, relieves gas, helps toothache, and treats menstrual cramps. As an expectorant and bronchodilator, clears mucus from the respiratory system.

*continued*

**L-TRYPTOPHAN** Anti-depressant. Sleep aid.

**UVA URSI** *(Arctostaphylos uva-ursi)* Diuretic, urinary antiseptic, astringent.

**VALERIAN** *(Valeriana officinalis)* Tranquilizer with few side effects. Aids sleep and helps fatigue.

**WINTERGREEN** *(Gaultheria procumbens)* Essential oil contains 90% methyl salicylate. Used in balms and ointments for arthritis, sciatica, and muscle spasm.

**WITCH HAZEL** *(Hamamelis virginiana)* Contains tannic acid, which helps stem bleeding of nosebleeds and cuts. Skin soother with pleasant odor.

**YARROW** *(Achillea millefolium)* Anti-spasmodic and astringent action useful in diarrhea and dysentery. Anti-inflammatory for arthritis and as an antiseptic.

## *READINGS

1. Gaby, A., & Wright, J. (1990). *Nutritional therapy for the 1990's.* Baltimore, MD: The Wright/Gaby Nutrition Institute.
2. Murray, M. (1994). *Natural alternatives.* New York: William Morrow.
3. Tyler, V. (1993). *The honest herbal.* Bingham, NY: The Hawarth Press.

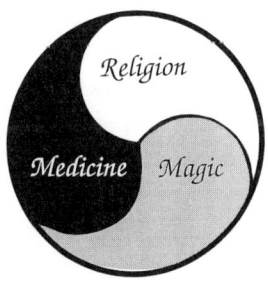

# IX

# DIET AND VITAMINS

ALTHOUGH HUNGER, starvation, and malnutrition are still worldwide problems, the focus on dietary considerations among affluent populations has turned toward an effort to change diets that are too rich, too caloric, too high in fat and cholesterol, and at the same time, too low in fiber. Evolutionary medicine points out that in the 10,000 years since humans began practicing agriculture, there has been only 0.005% change in our genes. Thus, a mismatch exists between the genetically determined physical and psychological needs of humans and their current environment. Four million years ago, our ancestors survived by eating plants. We are well adapted for such a diet. Unlike carnivores, we do not have fangs; like herbivores, we have molars for grinding. Although we cannot set back the clock of civilization, we can change personal life-styles that have led to the current epidemic of hypertension, cancer, and obesity.

**The Obesity Problem**

Many persons are struggling with the problem of obesity, but Albert Stunkard, M.D. (1), director of the Eating Disorders Clinic at the University of Pennsylvania, states that the belief that "fatness in general is bad for you" has been overrated. He points out that a level of 50% overweight raises the mortality rate by only 1.5%. Persons with upper-body obesity — apple shapes — suffer most of the medical complications. Such obesity is composed of fairly large fat cells. These abdominal cells make up high visceral fat and are the ones that do the damage. Men with pot bellies and high visceral fat are most in need of help. Obese women tend to have fat around the hips and thighs, and are pear-shaped. Composed of smaller fat cells, this type of obesity carries a lower medical risk. Such complications of obesity as high blood pressure, hyperlipidemia, hyperuricemia, and diabetes can be prevented and ameliorated by proper diet. Just taking off 10-15 pounds can help. Most persons set their goals at a far higher figure.

Despite the fact that 50% of American women and 25% of men have succumbed to the advertisements of highly touted schemes for reducing, there is no such thing as a "weight-loss diet"! Followed for a year, 95% of the patients are back to their old weight or even more. The "yo-yo effect" — going on and off diets with oscillating weight — is more harmful to the body than remaining at one level of weight. There is substantial evidence that obesity is a metabolic disorder: eating behavior and the regulation of body weight are carefully controlled physiological systems in human beings. Even obese persons are usually weight-stable. With successive "starvings," the body's metabolism can shift into low gear and develop a new set point for weight level. Hence, it is extremely difficult to slip below a temporary 15% reduction.

There is no secret or magical way to lose weight. Whatever calories are taken into the body must be entirely burned up or the excess will be stored as fat. For this reason, exercise is the vital component in any program to maintain or to lose weight. The correct approach to weight loss is simply a normal healthful diet but with a reduced number of calories. Added to this must be a program of increased activity.

Frank (2) eloquently discusses the role of the physician in the treatment of obesity. He points out that endorphins and serotonin levels regulate eating behavior and thermoregulation controls the dissipation of excess calories. Thus, weight level is a complex body process involving neurochemical, gastrointestinal, humoral, and genetic factors, as well as the autonomic nervous system. Yet this control can at times be overridden by a patient's deliberate behavior. This accounts for the widespread erroneous belief that obesity is simply a psychological problem characterized by a lack of willpower. Increasingly, physicians are coming to realize that obesity and over-eating are not the same. For too long, physicians have looked upon obesity as a social problem and have systematically avoided or given the treatment of obese patients short shrift. Granted, the treatment of obesity is difficult, most often goals are not reached, and the condition is chronic. But so is much of medicine. We don't abandon our diabetic patients because we can't cure them. It, too, is a chronic illness with complicated metabolic factors. Most physicians turn away from treating obese patients, rationalizing that obesity is a behavioral rather than a medical problem, and believing deep down that it is the patient's own fault. And so patients gravitate to commercial programs and practitioners of unconventional medicine. Book publishers, manufacturers of dietary nostrums, and well-advertised weight-loss schemes and clinics prosper. At any given time, an estimated 65 million Americans diet to lose weight, many consuming over-the-counter products or participating in weight-loss programs (3). Such programs may recommend very low calorie diets (800 calories per day) and rely heavily on behavioral modification such as teaching patients to recognize which situations and stimuli lead to food intake.

There is also interest in so-called "mood foods." Carbohydrates, for example, produce a calming effect on some persons. This is apparently related to serotonin activity. High-protein snacks, on the other hand, release dopamine and norepinephrine, which have been termed "alertness chemicals." Other researchers claim that taste is more addictive than either calories or nutrients, i.e., "the brain is more interested in what is happening on the tongue than in the stomach." (4)

The treatment of obesity has become a lucrative business. Many diets and fads come and go. Patients who go on diets, if followed a year later, are found to weigh the same as when they started the program. Such fad weight diets are usually some "food doctor's" promotion scheme based on a stated belief that adding or subtracting some items from the diet will bring about the desired weight loss. Some of the diets that have had popular acclaim are listed below. Some have no acceptable scientific backing, and while some are helpful, others can be harmful.

> **The Atkin's diet.** The basic idea here is that with a near-zero carbohydrate intake, hundreds of calories will leave the body every day in the form of ketones. This diet is not entirely safe, as the intake of cholesterol and saturated fats may be increased to a dangerous level.
>
> **Berger's immune power diet ("The Southampton Diet").** Recommends the eating of only "happy foods," which produce an elevation of "positive" neurotransmitters in the brain, as opposed to foods that produce elevation in "negative" neurotransmitters. While

immunologists rate food allergy as occurring in no more than 5% of persons, Berger states that everyone suffers from food allergy.

**Beverly Hills Diet.** Based on the idea that if certain specified foods are eaten in combination there will be an undigested food residue that accumulates and turns to fat.

**The Hay Diet.** Popular in the 30's, this was based on the principle of acid/base balance. Certain food combinations were recommended that are 20% acid-forming and 80% alkali-forming to produce a neutral condition in the body. This was felt to avoid successive episodes of constipation and diarrhea.

**Bircher-Benner System.** Diet used in the famous Zurich clinic established in 1902. The menu includes no meat, and consists mainly of raw foods, green leaves, lacto-ovarian protein, and whole grains. Aromatic herbs are used instead of condiments.

**Macrobiotics.** Popular in the 60's, this diet was derived from philosophical concepts of Traditional Chinese Medicine. Its founder, George Ohsawa, advocated the harmful practice of going for weeks eating nothing but brown rice. A recent version promoted by Michio Kushi includes a safer diet. The principle is to balance foods that are classed as *yin* (e.g., sugar, tofu, green vegetables, nuts, seeds, citrus fruits, and honey), with those classed as *yang* (e.g., meat, root vegetables, fish, beans, peas, and eggs). Brown rice and other whole grains are neutral and hence make up a good portion of the diet. Macrobiotic diets may resemble recommendations of the U.S. Surgeon General in that they usually are low in fat, cholesterol, and calories, and high in vegetables and fiber.

**Dean Ornish's diet.** Dr. Ornish, a cardiologist, has recommended a primarily vegetarian diet. His particular concern is that the average American eats eight times the needed amount of fat and cholesterol-containing foods. As the body manufactures its own cholesterol in sufficient quantities, cholesterol-containing foods are unnecessary and are to be avoided. As oils are liquid fats, he recommends that they be used with care. This diet has wide acceptance.

Persons from other parts of the world — Japan for example — who have diets low in fat have low blood pressure and lower rates of heart disease. Some fat, however, is essential in every diet. It is a source of the fat-soluble vitamins D,E,A, and K, and of the essential linoleic acid.

Dietary guidelines of the National Research Council (NRC) (5), which previously focused on overt clinical deficiencies, have more recently been concerned with dietary fat and cholesterol, which are predictors not only of coronary heart disease but also of cancer (6). These NRC recommendations (Table I) came about from observations of the relationship of total fat, saturated fat, and cholesterol blood levels to the clinically reported incidence of coronary heart disease (CHD). Recently, it has been shown that the blood level of high-density lipoprotein (HDL) cholesterol is inversely related to CHD and is a better predictor of heart problems than total cholesterol. Substitution of mono- or polyunsaturated fat in place of saturated fat reduces low density lipoprotein (LDL) levels without appreciably lowering HDL levels.

**Trans-fatty acids** are formed by the partial hydrogenation of liquid vegetable oils in the production of margarine and vegetable shortening. Intake of these foods has increased from zero percent in 1990 to now 5.5% of total fat and can account for up to 40% of dietary fat in the United States. In contrast, the amount of animal fat has decreased (6). Mono-unsaturated canola and olive oil are best. Next best are the poly-unsaturated fats, safflower and corn oil.

High intake of omega-3-fatty acids found in oils of fatty cold-water fish has accounted for a decreased incidence of heart disease in studies of fishermen from Greenland, and Japan. Research on intake of such fish oils indicates that they contain eicosapentanoic (EPA) and docosahexanoic (DHA) acids. These are found especially in salmon, sturgeon, and red snapper. Sardines, while very high in total omega-3 oils, are also relatively high in cholesterol.

Another omega-3-fatty acid is linolenic acid (LA), found in such foods as soybean oil, tofu, linseed and rapeseed oils, purslane, and seaweed. Linoleic (omega-6-fatty acid) is found in many vegetable oils but is less potent, having only two double bonds as compared to three to six in the omega-3 group.

## Is There an Anti-Cancer Diet?

There is increasing evidence that dietary fat is related to the development of breast, colon, and prostate cancer (6). The difference of increase in breast cancer between women in the United States versus women in Greece and Japan is as much as five-fold. Other factors which may also contribute to these differences are: reproductive patterns, physical activity, adiposity, alcohol intake, and the use of exogenous estrogens.

A positive association exists between animal (but not vegetable) fat and the incidence of colon cancer (6). This is especially true with red meat consumption and could relate to iron availability and heat-induced carcinogens. Such meat consumption has also been proposed as a factor in cancer of the prostate.

In addition to the recommendations to reduce the intake of animal fats, particularly from red meat, the intake of partially hydrogenated vegetable fat and saturated fat from dairy products should also be minimized. Evidence from epidemiological studies strongly suggests the importance of a generous intake of vegetables and fruits. Persons consuming higher amounts of these foods or having higher levels of carotenoids in their blood were less prone to develop cancer of the lung, stomach, breast, oral cavity, larynx, pancreas, bladder, and cervix (4). Colon cancer has an added risk factor of lower levels of folic acid and low fiber intake. It is associated with a higher intake of refined carbohydrates (i.e. white flour and sugar), which also lead to chronic diverticular diseases.

There is evidence that a good diet that avoids toxins and presumably boosts the immune system is important in the prevention of cancer. The National Cancer Institute is exploring the anti-cancer properties of phytochemicals that give plants protection against fungal and bacterial infections. These are particularly prominent in onions, garlic, carrots, celery, parsley, citrus fruits, and soybeans. Some work suggests that protection against breast cancer may be obtained by plants rich in indoles such as cabbage, brussels sprouts, and the cruciferous vegetables, cauliflower and broccoli. Emphasis is placed upon dark green, leafy vegetables — romaine in preference to iceberg lettuce, for example — and yellow foods, especially plenty of carrots.

Commonly recommended, especially by holistic practitioners, is that vitamin augmentation should include the anti-oxidant vitamins C, E, and A in the form of beta-carotene, together with the mineral supplement selenium. Support of this recommendation is not, however, universal. Herbert (7) has pointed out that some antioxidant vitamins are actually "redox" agents, acting sometimes as antioxidant and sometimes pro-oxidant. In RDA amounts and balanced biochemistry, the many redox and non-redox chemicals tend to be anti-oxidant. Above the RDA, he states, they unbalance biochemistry and tend to be pro-oxidant, thus increasing the risk of heart disease, cancer, and liver and kidney disease. Therefore, exceed RDA only with caution. Recent studies also suggest that high doses of beta carotene may increase the risk of cancer in smokers.

## TABLE V

### SUMMARY: DIETARY RECONSIDERATIONS NATIONAL RESEARCH COUNCIL

**Fat intake** under 30% or less of calories. Saturated fat intake less than 10% of calories and cholesterol less than 300 mg daily.

Five or more servings of **vegetables and fruits.** Emphasis on green and yellow vegetables and citrus fruits. Six or more servings of starches, grains and complex carbohydrates (breads, cereals, and legumes).

Maintain **protein intake** at moderate levels.

**Food intake and exercise** should balance for optimal body weight.

**Alcohol consumption** not recommended.

Total **salt intake** 6 grams or less.

Adequate **calcium intake.**

**Vitamins and minerals** at RDA levels, not above.

Optimal **fluoride intake** especially during years of growth and tooth formation.

# Diet and Vitamins

**Vitamins and Minerals**

Vitamins are organic substances that are essential in minute amounts for nutrition. They act as coenzymes or precursors of coenzymes necessary for the breakdown and metabolism of foods taken into the body. Minerals are also essential for metabolism and may act in conjunction with vitamins.

Vitamin/mineral supplements are taken by many persons, although some physicians believe this is unnecessary, for as they say, "with a good diet, one can obtain all that is required by the body." Unfortunately, people today live lives of stress, tend to skip meals, and rely on fast-food restaurants. Many foods today are processed, refined, and doctored with preservatives. Transit time from garden to plate is often prolonged. As foods are shipped from many parts of the world, they grow old and lose some of their nutrient value prior to consumption. For such reasons, supplementation with a multi-vitamin/mineral preparation is often good preventive medicine.

As vitamins are considered food, they are not under surveillance by the FDA. One should purchase only from a reliable manufacturer and be sure they are shelf-fresh and that all of the essential vitamins and minerals are present in the formulation.

Vitamins are commonly listed in terms of the percentage of the U.S. RDA (Recommended Daily Allowance), as determined by the National Academy of Science. Given either in units or milligram amounts, this percentage is the highest amount that should be taken on a daily basis. Vitamins and minerals must be obtained either from food in the diet or by supplementation because, with the exception of D and K, the body cannot make its own vitamins which therefore must be obtained from the diet.

It has been demonstrated that animals getting less than the RDA may develop symptoms known to occur with a deficiency of that particular vitamin or mineral. This has been the standard of vitamin and mineral recommendation for humans. However, as these data were determined from animal deprivation experiments, they are not always pertinent to humans. Observations of symptoms from humans with known vitamin deficiencies is a better standard. This is not readily accomplished, because apparently there are wide differences between humans in the amount of vitamins and minerals that may be required or tolerated.

Much confusion continues over the question of vitamin and mineral supplementation. Because vitamins are unregulated non-prescription items, they can simply be purchased by anyone, over the counter. The public has been led to believe that there is a general lack of vitamins, and hence, they have been added to many food products, including milk, breakfast cereals, candy bars, etc. The sale of vitamins is a lucrative business. They are advertised for their curative powers, even though many such claims are without scientific backing. Such advertising accounts for the overwhelming number of vitamin preparations seen on pharmacy and grocery store shelves. "Natural" vitamins are advertised at higher prices, as though they were superior to synthetic vitamins. There is, however, no discernible difference, as both the natural and the synthesized types are produced by chemical reactions and the final protein products as utilized by the body have identical chemical formulae.

Vitamins D, E, A, and K are fat-soluble and may be stored in the body over long periods of time. Thus, if taken in more than the recommended dose, they can collect in toxic amounts. Excess of vitamin D can cause improper deposition of calcium in the tissues and has been reputed to predispose to kidney stones. Vitamins E and A in excess can cause severe headaches, nausea, and other symptoms. Vitamin C and the B vitamins are water soluble and readily eliminated in urine and sweat and therefore are less likely to prove toxic. There are, however, limits above which their ingestion is not recommended. Vitamin B6, for example, was recently demonstrated to produce neurological symptoms if taken in excessive amounts. Large doses of vitamin C can produce diarrhea and a dependency state such that sudden withdrawal may produce the symptoms of scurvy. Niacin (vitamin B3) can produce severe flushing of the skin, pruritis, heart irregularity, liver toxicity, and other symptoms. Flushing is not seen when the amide form (niacinamide) is used in preference to niacin. Until more scientific, controlled experiments are available, a person could well expose himself to unknown risks if he consumes high doses of supplemental vitamins without proper supervision.

***Some Reputed Beneficial Effects of Vitamin Supplementation.*** Modern nutritionists believe that subclinical vitamin deficiencies may occur. Vitamin supplements may be helpful in such afflictions as minor skin irritations, small lesions about the lips, tongue, and eyes, increased susceptibility to infections, and slow healing of wounds. Special diets, increased stress, post-surgical operations, the use of cigarettes, alcohol, and caffeine, and problems associated with drug abuse may all significantly deplete vitamin stores. Requirements vary from person to person. Roger Williams, discoverer of pantothenic acid (vitamin B5) particularly emphasized the great variability in human physiology (8).

The term "megavitamin therapy," originating in the 1950's, refers to the use of large doses of vitamins for therapeutic purposes. Linus Pauling (9) used the term "Orthomolecular Medicine" in the 1960's to describe his recommendations for large doses of vitamin C. The term "Orthomolecular Psychiatry" is used to describe a form of megavitamin therapy introduced in 1952 by Drs. Abram Hoffer and Humphrey Osmond (10,11) for the treatment of psychiatric disorders. Since then, vitamins B6, B2, folic acid, and others have also been used in mega-doses for such patients. The theory is that a well-nourished brain responds better to other therapies. Orthomolecular psychiatric treatment is still in need of further scientific study. A recent article by Barrett (12) reviews scientific literature which gives no support to the claims of benefit from large doses of vitamin C.

Various vitamin combinations have been suggested as curative for arthritic conditions. In addition to recommendations by Linus Pauling for as much as 5-10 grams of vitamin C as a daily supplement, vitamin B6 has been often suggested for such conditions (13).

Table VI gives the RDA of vitamins and minerals and an indication of mega-doses that have been recommended in the literature of Alternative Medicine. Table VII lists some recommendations that have been given for therapeutic uses of vitamin and mineral supplements.

## REFERENCES

1. Stunkard, A., & Wadden T. (Eds.). (1993). *Obesity, theory and therapy.* (2nd ed.). New York: Raven Press.
2. Frank, A. (1993). Futility and avoidance: Medical professionals in the treatment of obesity. *JAMA, 269,* 2132-2133.
3. Blackburn, G. (1993, January). Medical solutions to obesity. *Physician's Travel and Meeting Guide,* pp. 29-30.

4. Brown, N. (1993, January 17). Mind over munchies. *St. Louis Post Dispatch, PD Magazine,* p. 18.
5. National Research Council. (1989). *Diet and health: Implications for reducing chronic disease risk.* Washington, D.C.: National Academy Press.
6. Willett, W. (1994). Diet and health: What should we eat? *Science, 264,* 532-537.
7. Herbert, V. (1994). The antioxidant supplement myth. *Amer J Clin Nutr, 4,* 60-157.
8. Williams, Roger. (1977). *The wonderful world within you.* New York: Bantam Books.
9. Pauling, Linus. (1971). *Vitamin C and the common cold.* New York: Bantam Books.
10. Hoffer, A., & Osmond, H. (1966). *How to live with schizophrenia.* New Hyde Park, NY: University Books.
11. Pfeiffer, C. (1975). *Mental and elemental nutrients.* New Canaan, CT: Keats.
12. Barrett, S. (1995). The dark side of Linus Pauling's legacy. *Skeptical Inquirer, 19,* 18-20.
13. Ellis, J. (1971). *The doctor who looked at hands.* New York: RC Books.

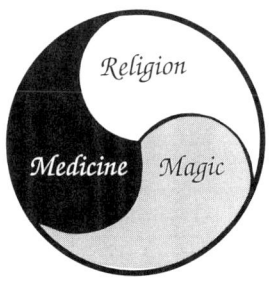

# TABLE VI

## DOSE SCHEDULE OF VITAMINS AND MINERALS

### VITAMINS
RECOMMENDED DAILY REQUIREMENT

|  | RDA |  | MEGADOSE* | |
|---|---|---|---|---|
| A (retinal) (beta carotene) | 5,000 | I.U. | | |
| B1 (thiamine) | 2.5 | mg | 100-500 | mg |
| B2 (riboflavin) | 2.5 | mg | 10-75 | mg |
| B3 (niacin) | 30 | mg | 3 | Gm |
| B5 (pantothenic acid) | 15 | mg | 150 | mg |
| B6 (pyridoxine) | 3 | mg | 150-500 | mg |
| B12 (cyanocobalamine) | 9 | ug | 1000 | ug IM |
| C (ascorbic acid) | 250 | mg | 3-10 | Gm |
| D (calciferol) | 400 | I.U. | | |
| E (tocopherol) | 30 | I.U. | 200-800 | mg |
| K (menedine) | (20-25 | mg only if needed) | | |
| Biotin | 0.45 | mg | 300 | mg |
| Folic Acid | 0.4 | mg | 1-5 | mg |

### MAJOR MINERALS

| Calcium Chloride | 1 | Gm |
|---|---|---|
| Potassium | | |
| Magnesium | 600 | mg |
| Sodium | | |
| Phosphorus | 1.5 | Gm |

### TRACE ELEMENTS

| Cobalt | | | | |
|---|---|---|---|---|
| Chromium | 1 | mg | | |
| Copper | 2 | mg | | |
| Fluoride | | | | |
| Iron | 25 | mg | | |
| Iodine | 225 | ug | | |
| Manganese | 5 | mg | 6 | mg |
| Molybdenum | 0.1 | mg | | |
| Selenium | 0.2 | mg | | |
| Zinc | 20 | mg | 45 | mg |
| Choline | | | | |

### OTHER

| Linoleic acid | | | | |
|---|---|---|---|---|
| PABA (para-aminobenzoic acid) | 30 | mg | 1,200 | mg |
| Inositol 250 mg | | | 1 | Gm |
| Rutin | 50 | mg | 1 | Gm |
| Bioflavinoids | | | | |

"Vitamin P:" A mixture of substances obtained from various plant sources usually including citrin and bioflavonoids.

*Beware toxicity.

## TABLE VII

### VITAMIN USES THAT HAVE BEEN SUGGESTED BY SOME HOLISTIC PRACTITIONERS

**Thiamin (B1):** Anti-stress, neuralgia, various neurological diseases. Treatment of beri-beri.

**Riboflavin (B2):** In combination with B6 for carpal tunnel syndrome and related problems. This condition apparently occurs with a deficiency in EGOT (erythrocyte glutamic oxaloacetic transaminase), which is corrected by B6 (100 mg daily) and a deficiency in EGT (erythrocyte glutamic reductase), which is corrected by Riboflavin (50 mg daily).

**Niacin (B3):** For elevated cholesterol. Treatment of alcoholism and in Orthomolecular psychiatry for schizophrenia, depression, and others. Treatment of pellagra.

**Pantothemic Acid (B5):** For allergy and as a cream for skin conditions.

**Pyridoxine (B6):** Carpal tunnel syndrome as above. Also premenstrual tension, migraine, and arthritis involving the hands. Hyperkinesis accompanying serotonin deficiency.

**Cyanocobalamine (B12):** Pernicious anemia. Given by hypodermic (1000 micrograms) for various neurological diseases.

**Folic Acid:** Psychiatric problems in the aged. Canker sores, gout, and psoriasis. Supplements to pregnant women can prevent occurrence of spina bifida and anencephaly.

**Biotin:** Eczema.

*continued*

**Ascorbic Acid (C):** Antioxidant in cancer prevention. Boosts immune function for prevention of virus and bacterial infections. Orthomolecular psychiatry in large doses for schizophrenia and alcoholism. Treatment of scurvy. Prevents cataracts. Reduced incidence of strokes.

**Retinal (A):** Acute infections, skin conditions. The water soluble precursor, beta-carotene, is an anti-oxidant useful in cancer prevention, although may increase risk of cancer in smokers. Prevents cataracts. Reduced incidence of strokes. Supplements prevent child mortality in developing countries.

**Calciferol (D):** Aids absorption of calcium. Useful with hormone administration to prevent osteoporosis.

**Tocopherol (E):** As anti-oxidant to prevent cancer. In fibrocystic breast disease. Cataract prevention. Cuts risk of heart and blood vessel disease (recommendation from the American Heart Association).

**Calcium:** Muscle cramps. With vitamin D for prevention of osteoporosis.

**Magnesium:** Asthma, fatigue, depression. (Reported in *JAMA* Nov. 4, 1992: to assist during heart surgery and reduce cardiac arrhythmia).

**Iron:** Iron deficiency anemia. Restless leg syndrome.

**Selenium:** As an antioxidant for prevention of cancer.

**Chromium:** Diabetes.

**Zinc:** Essential to the immune system — skin and virus infections. Prostate enlargement. Loss of taste and smell.

# X

# TRADITIONAL CHINESE AND NEURO-ELECTRIC ACUPUNCTURE

THIS CHAPTER presents an outstanding example of how the diligent and meticulous application of the principles of scientific research to a practice of alternative medicine can replace fanciful theories with factual explanations. Among the 50 or more unconventional practices under the heading of "alternative medicine," only a few have been demonstrated to have a truly scientific basis. Acupuncture is the one great exception. Perhaps some inquisitive minds will enlist the principles of scientific research to fill in the gaps of knowledge about other holistic procedures that may then become part of the treatment armamentarium of Western healers.

**Acupuncture**

It is increasingly common these days to learn of someone who has received "miraculous relief" from acupuncture for some condition of chronic pain that had not improved when treated with the usual methods of Western medicine. Headaches, backaches, sciatica, and post-herpetic neuralgia, along with a myriad of other conditions, have all responded well to acupuncture. Patients treated for drug and alcohol addiction have praised the pleasurable feelings of relaxation and return of body homeostasis produced when electrical stimulation is applied to acupuncture sites.

Just what is going on here? What is acupuncture really all about? For hundreds of years, the manner in which acupuncture produced its effects was shrouded in the Oriental mystery of metaphysics. Only in the last two decades, after scientists began to understand the intricate neurophysiology of the pain response, has a scientific interpretation of acupuncture become possible.

Today, many persons in various parts of the world still practice acupuncture according to traditional, centuries-old Chinese techniques. This may be because they have not been trained in the mode of scientific thinking characteristic of modern medicine or because they have not become acquainted with the results of recent scientific acupuncture research, much of it done in China. This could have given them the information needed to replace their outmoded ideas.

In order to better understand what is meant by the term "acupuncture," it will be necessary to review its ancient history and cosmological beginnings before proceeding to explain in scientific terms how acupuncture really works.

### Ancient Acupuncture (1)

While modern medicine deals with known anatomical and physiological facts about body structures, classical Chinese medicine deals with functions to which actual body organs are only incidentally attached.

In Chinese medicine, the practice of acupuncture is based on "*meridian* theory," a belief that body energies such as *ch'i* travel about the body in imaginary channels called *sinarteries* or *meridians*. Such *meridians* are hypothetical constructs and have no anatomic reality. Although the *meridians* themselves are only the result of speculation, they serve as a useful mnemonic method in Traditional Chinese Acupuncture for remembering the placement of needles. Kim Bong Han of Korea, using microdissection, found fine tubules which he called *meridians*. Others have failed to verify this. More recently, Pierre de Vernejoul of France, using radioactive isotopes, felt that he could distinguish "*meridian* channels" from blood vessels and nerves. Apart from such isolated, non-replicated reports, contemporary physicians in Russia, Japan, China, and the West have tried in vain to prove the existence of such conduits. Such efforts fail to recognize that the concept of *meridians* is important only as an hypothetical construct invented for the support of a metaphysical theory involving the manipulation of *ch'i* by means of needles in acupuncture points. Believers in other unconventional healing methods that lack any proven scientific basis have attributed great physiological significance to *ch'i* and to these imaginary conduits, and have used the *meridian* concept to support arcane beliefs such as reflexology, tongue diagnosis, and *chakras*.

In Traditional Chinese Medicine, there are twelve paired and two unpaired *meridians* (Table VIII). There are, in addition, a number of accessory *meridians* of less importance.

## TABLE VIII
### THE TRADITIONAL ACUPUNCTURE MERIDIANS

| | |
|---|---|
| LI-LARGE INTESTINE | LU-LUNG |
| BL-BLADDER | KI-KIDNEY |
| GB-GALL BLADDER | LI-LIVER |
| SP-SPLEEN | ST-STOMACH |
| SI-SMALL INTESTINE | HT-HEART |
| TH-TRIPLE HEATER | PC-PERICARDIUM |

### UNPAIRED MERIDIANS

GV-GOVERNING VESSEL
CV-CONCEPTION VESSEL

Acupuncture is only one part of Traditional Chinese Medicine, but it is the part that has received the greatest attention in the West. It consists of placing small steel needles in spots on the skin designated as "acupuncture points." These needles are then manipulated in various ways in order to control the flow of the presumed body energy, *ch'i*. Originally, cosmologically, with reference to the days of the year, there were 362 acupuncture points. These were thought to be spots where body energy came close to the surface of the skin. It was believed that such points were small hollow areas (*hsueh*). As persons varied in size, these points were located by measuring distances from anatomical landmarks such as bony protuberances. The distance between two creases on the patient's flexed middle finger was used as a ruler. This was their *chun*, their own "body inch" (Figure 5).

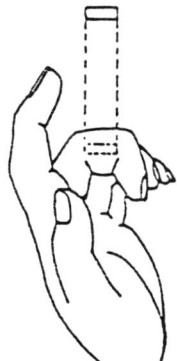

**Figure 5. The *chun* or body inch.**

Once these *meridian* lines had been hypothesized, succeeding generations of acupuncturists felt free to find and arbitrarily describe special acupuncture points along these hypothesized conduits designated according to the discoverer's belief. Thus, today there are over 1000 described points covering almost every part of the body. Modern researchers have found that of these many points, only about 80 are useful and have a physiological significance, being either motor points or points near Golgi tendon organs or near important nerve structures.

In the metaphysical belief of Traditional Chinese Medicine, illness is conceived as an imbalance of *Yin* and *Yang*, the two fundamental opposing forces of polarity that exist in all of nature. The goal of treatment by acupuncture is to correct this imbalance.

In early China was the belief that the world was composed of several elemental substances: wood, fire, earth, water, and metal. The so-called "five element theory" was concerned with the interactions, combinations, and seemingly endless intertwining of these basic substances that composed the universe. As diagrammed (Figure 6), these elements succeed each other in a circular order. Moving clockwise, the sequence becomes the "evolutive or productive" phase. Moving around the circle in a counter-clockwise direction, the elements can also be thought of as having the ability to check or modify each preceding element in turn. As

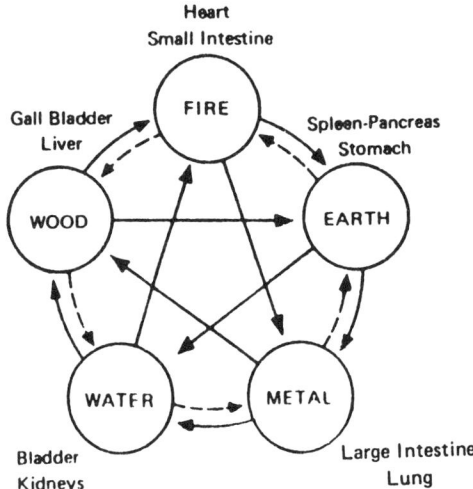

Figure 6. The five elements (essences) with their corresponding organs, illustrating how these essences interact and influence one another.

each element is related to or represents two body organs, the stimulation by acupuncture of those points on a *meridian* representing one set of organs is believed to influence the behavior or function of two other organs related to another element. Disturbances of body function or illnesses are thought of in terms of "deficiencies" or "excesses," which can occur through the influence of one element overpowering another, as illustrated by its position on the circular diagram. This is known as "The Law of Wu Hing," in which the clockwise direction is called the *Sheng* Cycle, while counter-clockwise it is the *Ko* Cycle (Table IX).

The procedure of pulse diagnosis is designed to determine the strength, weakness, or disturbance in the various organ systems. After such diagnosis is made by distinguishing 27 varieties of pulse at six different locations on each of the two wrists, the acupuncturist proceeds to determine which *meridians* and points to stimulate by following the "Law of Wu Hing."

This, then, is a very simplistic explanation for the climatic, macrocosmic influences on the physiology of the body that make up the hypothetical understructure upon which were based the diagnosis and acupuncture treatment procedures of Traditional Chinese Medicine.

## TABLE IX

### DOCTRINE OF THE FIVE ELEMENTS
### "THE LAW OF WU HING"

*Illustrating How These Elements Exercise an Influence Upon One Another*

**THE SHENG CYCLE**

FIRE engenders EARTH
EARTH engenders METAL
METAL engenders WATER
WATER engenders WOOD
WOOD engenders FIRE

**THE KO CYCLE**

FIRE overcomes METAL by melting
METAL overcomes WOOD by cutting
WOOD overcomes EARTH by covering
EARTH overcomes WATER by damming
WATER overcomes FIRE by extinguishing

---

In addition to placement of the needle in the proper point on the indicated *meridian*, additional strength is supposed to be given to the treatment by the burning of a pellet of moxa on the needle. This is termed "moxabustion." The substance burned is wormwood *(artemesia absinthium)*, which can be placed either on the needle or burned on a slip of ginger root placed on the skin. In some cases, burning moxa "cigars" are held directly over or against the skin but always at the proper acupuncture points.

Because of its many ramifications and interdependencies, Chinese medicine is so complex that it is said to take a lifetime for its complete mastery. Such mastery of traditional Chinese acupuncture is not necessary to equip one to practice modern scientific acupuncture (neuroelectric acupuncture or NEAP). It only prepares one to practice the age-old cult of Traditional Chinese Folk Medicine. Research from around the world has now added scientific knowledge which makes traditional acupuncture an obsolete practice. It is to the credit of Chinese researchers that their persistence in pursuing studies of both animal models and clinical patients has resulted in the modern practice of NEAP.

**Scientific Developments Leading to Neuro-Electric Acupuncture (NEAP)**

The popularity of acupuncture has waxed and waned over the centuries. By the year **500** C.E., it had spread to Korea and Japan and was introduced to France and other European countries by missionaries in the **1700's**. In **1882** in China, it was banned by the Emperor as an impediment to medical progress and removed from the curriculum of the Imperial Medical College. It was again popularized in the **1940's** by Maoists faced with a paucity of well-trained physicians as a means to supply some type of medical treatment to China's millions. In the U.S. in **1912**, a book by famed Johns Hopkins professor William Osler, *Principles and Practices of Medicine,* recommended acupuncture for the treatment of sciatica. In subsequent editions of this book, the reference to acupuncture was deleted and acupuncture was virtually unknown in the U.S. until **1972**.

When acupuncture was reintroduced to America at the time of President Nixon's visit to China, U.S. physicians visited China and witnessed surgery done without chemical anesthesia, with only electro-acupuncture analgesia. They were unable to accept explanations in terms of the *Yin/Yang* and *meridian* theories. They concluded that acupuncture was a form of "Oriental hypnosis." In **1972**, the American Medical Association branded acupuncture an "experimental procedure," and 20 years later, despite increasing scientific evidence to the contrary, the AMA's position has not changed.

With much publicity, acupuncture was promoted in the Western world as a "cure-all." When it was rejected by organized medicine, non-medical persons moved to meet the demand that arose for this treatment. Today, persons with no medical knowledge can take a 200-hour course in what is essentially Chinese metaphysics and, in many countries and over half the states in the U.S., become certified for what is actually the "practice of medicine" by persons without medical training.

Our group at the University of Missouri received the first grant given by the National Institutes of Health to compare acupuncture and hypnosis for the relief of pain (**1972**). We used healthy volunteers exposed to experimental pain produced by both cold pressor (water bath) and electric shock. We compared the protective effects of hypnosis, 10 mg of morphine sulfate given intra-muscularly, and acupuncture. The last was administered with needles inserted at both specific (acupuncture) and nonspecific (placebo) points, with and without electrical stimulation.

In **1976**, we published results showing that acupuncture was not hypnosis and that while needles alone produced some treatment effect, electrical stimulation of the needles was necessary for a significant relief of pain (2) (Figure 7). Work of Liu et al. in **1975** (3) and Gunn in **1977** (4) convinced us that *meridians* did not exist and that of the traditional 362 acupuncture points, there are only about 80 important ones, including motor points and points near major nerves. It is also interesting that the painful "*ah shi*" (in Chinese, "oh yes") points of acupuncture are actually the tender muscle trigger points described in the American literature by Travell (5).

In **1965**, Melzack and Wall (6) suggested how the control of pain might occur. This was their famous "gate theory," in which they demonstrated that the nerves carrying pain impulses could be blocked by stimulation of a different system of nerves. Such stimulation, they said, "closed the gate on pain." In **1973**, Pert and Snyder (7) demonstrated that there were opiate receptors on nerve cells, spots where substances like opium and other "pain killing" drugs could act to relieve pain. In **1975**, Kosterlitz and Hughes (8) wrote about the significance of inner secretions, the body's own "pain killers," opiate-like substances named "endorphins," meaning endogenous (body-produced) morphine. In **1977**, Mayer (9) demonstrated the significance of a compound that could halt the action of opiate compounds. This was called "naloxone." Sjolund, Terenius, and Erickson (10) demonstrated in **1977** that endorphins are increased in cerebrospinal fluid with electro-acupuncture stimulation. Peets and Pomeranz reported in **1978** (11) that a strain of mice deficient in opiate receptors showed a poor response to electro-acupuncture given to produce an analgesic control of pain.

In **1987**, Professor Ji Sheng Han of Beijing Medical University published *The Neurochemical Basis of Pain Relief by Acupuncture* (12).

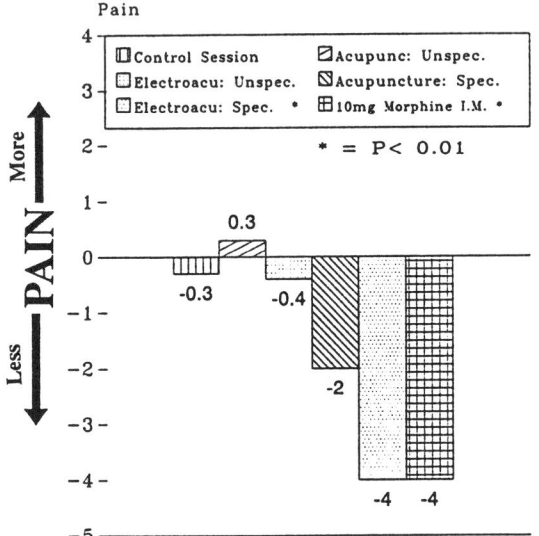

Figure 7. Changes in subjective experience of experimental pain with different pain challengers. Demonstrates the importance of electrical stimulation (20 subjects).

This landmark volume was a review of 120 studies from his laboratory demonstrating the various chemicals in the brain that are important for the control of pain. These studies began after observations of surgical patients receiving acupuncture analgesia, where it was noted that with continued electrical stimulation, the pain threshold continued to rise over a 30-minute period and returned gradually to the pre-stimulation level when the electrical stimulation of the acupuncture needles was stopped. This prompted experiments involving the cross-infusion of cerebrospinal fluid in animals. Here it was observed that when cerebrospinal fluid from an animal that had developed electro-acupuncture analgesia was injected into a non-stimulated animal, there was a similar but smaller analgesic reaction. This showed that the electro-acupuncture stimulation had produced a chemical change in the cerebrospinal fluid of the stimulated animal, which was transferred into the non-stimulated animal, thus producing a rise in the pain threshold.

A most important development occurred in **1990** when Han (13) reported that electrical stimulation of acupuncture points, using different frequencies of stimulation, produced the release of different neuropeptides in the central nervous system. Stimulation at slow frequencies (two cycles per second) caused a rise in endorphins. Faster frequencies produced the release of other neuropeptides. For example, 15 cycles per second released enkephalins, while 100 cycles per second released dynorphins (Figure 8). These neuropeptides, important for the transmission of nervous impulses in the brain, produced not only significant pain control but also other changes in the nervous system that brought about feelings of well-being and relief from depression. These compounds, then, are the body's own opioids and have certain features in common with the exogenous opioid group of drugs, e.g., heroin and morphine.

The above shows that which frequency of electrical stimulation is used is far more important than where the needles are placed. Han compared the use of electrically stimulated acupuncture needles with conducting polymer pad electrodes. He used different frequencies of stimulation and found that with all frequencies studied, the pads produced just as good pain control as the needles. Thus, it can be concluded that for pain control, it is essential to use electrical stimulation, that the frequency of stimulation is important, that the points stimulated should be motor points where nerve enters muscle, and that needles are no longer essential.

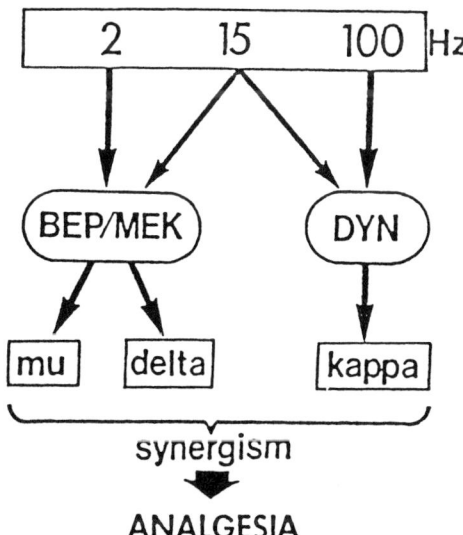

Figure 8. Electro-acupuncture at different frequencies of stimulation releases different kinds of neuropeptides in the central nervous system. These act upon different types of opiate receptors on cells of the CNS (mu—B-endorphins, delta—met-enkephalins, kappa—dynorphins).

There is a saying in China that one generation builds the road upon which another generation travels. That was certainly true in the development of modern electro-acupuncture with its effect upon pain and behavior through the release of important brain chemicals. How prophetic were the words of Chairman Mao when he said, "Ancient Chinese Medicine is a veritable storehouse."

And what of ear acupuncture? Traditional Chinese acupuncturists believed that the various *meridians* of the body began, ended in, or traversed the ear. Dr. Nogier, a French acupuncturist, expanded upon this belief and promoted it under the name "auriculotherapy." (14)

Charts of the ear show all parts of the body on a map appearing like "an embryo upside down" with the head at the lower end of the ear (Figure 9). Some 168 points are described on this ear map of the body. However, there is no anatomical proof that a map of the body should appear on the surface of the ear. Such belief is like that of reflexologists who believe that a map of the body exists on the sole of the foot, or of *Koryo* Hand Acupuncturists who treat all illnesses by stimulating "body points" on the hand. In a controlled cross-over study, Melzac (15) found that ear acupuncture did not give pain relief beyond that of placebo.

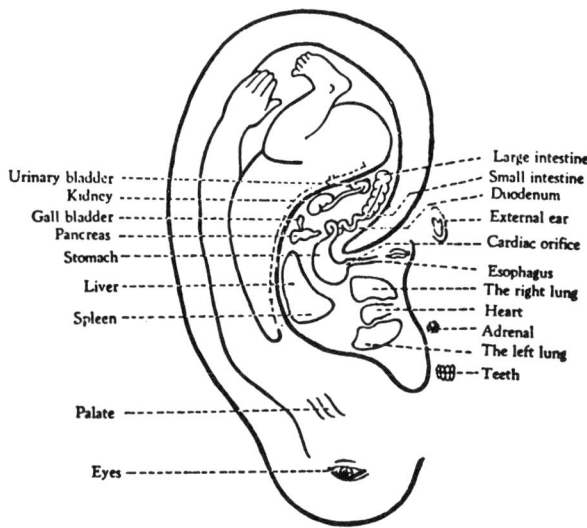

Figure 9. Basic diagram of Auriculotherapy. Corresponding representation of body areas to ear points resembling an "embryo upside down."

Such beliefs about ear acupuncture may have been strengthened by the fact that the vagus nerve innervates the hollow part, concha, of the ear (Figure 10). The vagus nerve represents an important part of the parasympathetic nervous system. While the sympathetic nervous system reacts to stress by producing increased activity throughout the whole body, i.e., rapid heart beat, higher blood pressure, tension in the gut, etc., the parasympathetic portion of the autonomic nervous system produces the opposite, a calming effect on all body organs. Thus, electrical stimulation at any part of the vagus (parasympathetic) area of the ear can bring about a homeostatic effect upon body viscera. It does this by affecting all organs as a group, but not point-by-point on an individual basis. Thus, there is no "body map" on the ear.

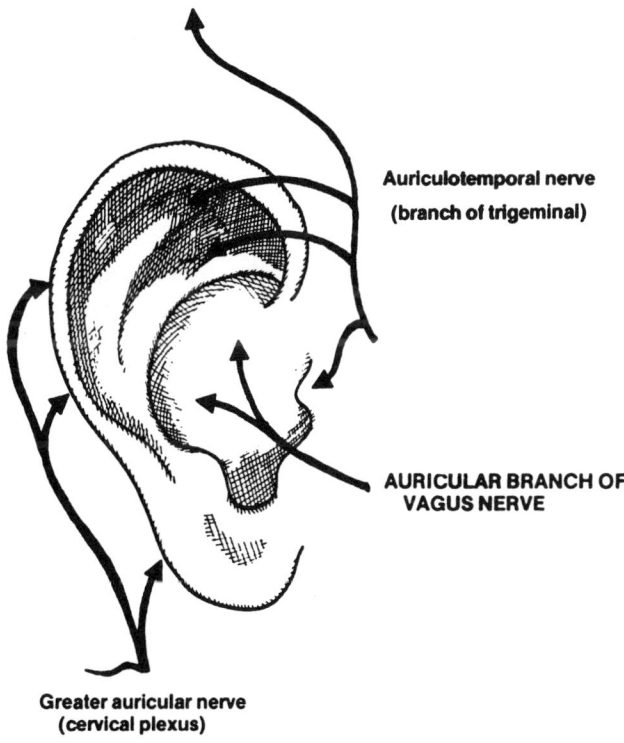

Figure 10. Innervation of the ear.

In **1972**, Dr. Wen of Hong Kong (16) showed that an electrically stimulated needle placed in the concha of the ear could help overcome the withdrawal symptoms of persons addicted to heroin. As withdrawal effects from heroin are characterized by symptoms of sympathetic over-reaction, it is understandable that vagus stimulation, with its parasympathetic, calming effect, could be helpful. Somehow, in ensuing years, people seem to have forgotten that Dr. Wen used electrical stimulation of the ear needles, and many clinics today are treating addiction in the old-fashioned manner of auriculotherapy by simply inserting a number of unstimulated needles in the supposed body points of the ear. This would produce primarily a placebo effect.

**Pain**

*The Nature of Pain.* Pain causes endless suffering, alters lives, frustrates health care providers, and costs untold billions of dollars in medical procedures, pills, and time lost from work. Despite the great advances in medical science, efforts to control chronic pain are often ineffectual. For millions of patients and their families, chronic pain and suffering produces severe physical, social, and emotional consequences.

Yet pain is one of the essential bodily sensations. Without the ability to feel pain, we could not remain alive for long. Very rarely, children are born without a thalamus, that portion of the brain in which pain is experienced. Such children do not feel burns or injuries and quickly succumb to resultant bleeding and infections. Thus, pain has a very useful function.

For example, if you stumble out of bed in the middle of the night and bump your toe, you experience pain. The pain impulse travels up the nerves of the leg, up the spinal cord to the thalamus where pain is experienced.

At this point, one knows only that there has been an injury, but not where. Beyond the thalamus, the impulse travels to the top of the brain. Here, in the sensory area of the cerebral cortex, is a map of the body sometimes called the *homunculus* or "little man." Here, you learn that it is your toe that has been injured. You then reach down and rub the skin of your toe. This is "pain behavior." The pleasant massage from rubbing the skin excites the pain control nervous network that modulates or blocks pain impulses. If the pain goes away, it has served its useful purpose of alerting the therapist to the area of tissue damage.

If, despite continuing massage of the toe, the pain continues day after day and week after week, you experience "useless" or chronic pain. In this instance, the second portion of the pain nervous system, the part that modulates or blocks pain, has not worked properly. Thus, there are two parts of the pain nervous system: one that turns pain "on" and one that turns pain "off." Were it not so, we would all be in misery all of our lives, for hardly a day goes by that one does not experience some small injury with accompanying pain sensation, minor though it may be.

We now know that the second anti-pain part of the nervous system is activated by chemicals called neuropeptides. Dr. Bruce Pomeranz of Toronto, Canada, (11) bred a strain of rats in which the chemicals responsible for the modulation of pain were deficient. Perhaps the small number of patients who fail to react well to acupuncture are similarly deficient.

*Pain and the Nervous System.* To understand the workings of the nervous system, it is basic to realize that the nerve cells do not conduct nervous impulses as though they were continuous wires. Nerve cells are separated from each other by very minute spaces called synapses. The nervous impulse must cross this space for communication from one cell to another. The ability to cross this space is controlled by certain chemicals called neuro-regulators. These play a key role in the communication between nerve cells. There are two types of such neuroregulators, the neurotransmitters that carry the information forward, and the neuromodulators that either amplify or dampen the message.

The discovery of the opioid receptor sites on nerve cells was important for an understanding of how pain is regulated. These receptors are binding sites on the membranes of cells that transmit and modulate pain impulses. There are at least three kinds of substances important for conducting pain impulses. These are the neuropeptides—Beta-endorphin, methionine and leucine enkephalin, and dynorphin. These are known as "opiate agonists," as they act on the nerve cells in the fashion of opium or morphine. Substances that block this action and thus increase pain are called "opiate antagonists." The best known of these is naloxone.

The arcuate nucleus of the hypothalamus gives rise to pro-opiomelanocortin, which is the mother molecule of the opioids. Not only acupuncture, but TENS, pain, damaged tissue, and physical activity give rise to this substance. By activation, this precursor, pro-opiomelancortin, is split into three major bioactive neuropeptide fractions: adrenocorticotropin (ACTH), three variants of the melanocyte hormones, and B-endorphin.

The opioid peptides induce analgesia in several ways: *1)* by blocking pain impulses as they enter from the periphery into the dorsal horn region of the spinal cord; *2)* by blocking the transmission of pain impulses on their way upward to the brain at supra-spinal levels; and *3*) by stimulating higher neural mechanisms that send messages down to block pain at lower and spinal cord levels.

Another transmitter substance known as serotonin acts in the midbrain area and is also involved in producing analgesia. Both central serotonin and the endorphins regulate systems that can slow the pulse, lower blood pressure, and inhibit overaction of body organs. This, known as splanchnic activation, occurs after electro-acupuncture stimulation. It is interesting that this effect is more pronounced in persons who have hypertension and other bodily dysregulation. This is in keeping with the widespread belief that acupuncture produces a return to resting levels when the body homeostatic mechanisms are disturbed.

Evidence supporting the observation that electro-acupuncture can decrease pain by releasing an endogenous substance with opiate-like activity (endorphins, enkephalins, or dynorphins) is demonstrated by the fact that acupuncture analgesia in humans can be reversed by the endorphin blocker naloxone.

It is interesting that analgesia can also result from painful and stressful manipulations of the body. This type of noxious stimulation probably involves other pathways. Analgesia thus may come about by descending impulses in both opiate and non-opiate analgesic systems. Jogging and strong physical exercise have been commonly recognized as relieving chronic pain. This "jogger's high" probably occurs from stimulation of muscle afferents, and may involve the same nerve pathways that are stimulated by electro-acupuncture over points where nerves enter muscles. Psychiatrists have long considered depression to be one of the most painful of illnesses, and jogging and exercise are often part of programs designed to treat depression.

Pain can be controlled in several other ways. The surgical cutting of nerves can produce areas of local analgesia, but this is not a good way to control chronic pain because, as we have seen, pain involves the whole nervous system — spinal cord, lower brain centers, and cortex. Melzac and others have said that chronic pain is like a pain memory involving reverberating, self-sustaining neural circuits in the brain. This is well demonstrated by persons who have "phantom limb pain," which persists as a memory of an arm or leg after that limb has been amputated from the body. Control of such "phantom limb pain" by electro-acupuncture illustrates the importance of central pain control.

Most commonly, patients attempt to control pain by taking "pain pills." This is no cure, but simply gives temporary relief. Once taken, such pills must usually be continued over long periods of time with continuing expense. There are also many side effects that can occur with such medications. Thus, a non-pharmacological procedure like electro-acupuncture assumes great importance.

***Clinical Use of Acupuncture for Pain Control.*** Body electro-acupuncture is regularly reported to produce pain relief in 60-75% with various types of pain. This compares to 30-35% of pain relief in placebo controls as shown by Lewith et al. (17) Success has been reported from clinical use of TENS (18), thus illustrating again the importance of electrical stimulation.

Electro-acupuncture treatments for pain are usually given in the setting of the doctor's office. The patient lies comfortably on a couch. If needles are used, they should be of very fine diameter. Today, disposable needles are used so there is no danger of transferring infection from one patient to another. Because these needles are so fine and flexible, their insertion is assisted by means of a small plastic tube which is held against the skin, with the handle of the needles protruding 1/4 of an inch above the end of the tube (Figure 11). This end is given a tap so that the needle penetrates the skin without pain. The needle can then be twisted in to any desired depth. As it nears the nervous structures, there is usually a dull drawing sensation. The Chinese have called this *teh ch'i*, a "drawing of the *ch'i*." As it has been found that conducting polymer pad electrodes are equally as effective as needles, they are now more frequently used. With electrical stimulation, precise positioning is not essential, as the current can spread with increased intensity. In some applications, for anatomical reasons such as hairy areas, needles are preferable. In many cases, treatments are given using both needles and pad electrodes.

Electrical stimulation is used for all treatments, since it has been shown that electricity is the essential ingredient for clinical acupuncture. The frequency of the current used is important because specific frequencies release specific neuropeptides. Often, a so-called "Dense/Disperse" setting of the stimulator is used. In this setting, the current alternates between a slow frequency — two cycles per second, which releases endorphins — and a higher frequency, which releases enkephalins or dynorphins.

The optimal time for a treatment is 30 minutes. Treatments are usually given initially once or twice a week, although daily treatment may be indicated for acute conditions. As the patient improves, the interval between treatments is lengthened. Often, patients will obtain sufficient pain relief with only ten or twelve treatments. At times, a maintenance program is necessary, with treatments being continued on a monthly basis. Sometimes, patients will obtain complete relief with a few treatments but may find the pain later returns. Another session of a smaller number of treatments may produce lasting relief.

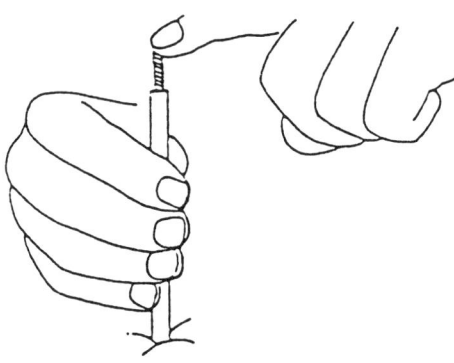

**Figure 11. Hollow tube method of inserting fine, disposable acupuncture needles.**

## Addiction

Addiction has been defined as the continual requirement for a particular substance in order to maintain a feeling of comfort. The essential features of an addictive drug are:

- Short-acting.
- Produces an elevation of mood or a euphoric effect.
- Tolerance develops with continued use, so that the amount of substance that has to be consumed to produce the same effect must be increased.
- Produces a withdrawal response, the features of which are peculiar to the individual drug and person.
- Invariably finally associated with adverse effects on physical and mental health; causes social problems.

The exogenous opioid morphine is an example of an addicting drug. Heroin, which is a very short-acting opioid, produces an elevation of mood. Tolerance develops rapidly, depending on the quality and the amount of the drug taken. These opioids are not the only important drugs of addiction. Nicotine, alcohol, the benzodiazepines (valium, librium, etc.), caffeine, amphetamines (dexedrine, etc.), cocaine, volatile substances that are sniffed, and others can all addict. The most commonly used drug of addiction with probably the longest history of abuse is alcohol.

Usually a person becomes addicted to one substance and uses this in preference to all others. In the history of an addict, however, there may have been a progression of use from teenage on, starting with cigarettes, progressing to alcohol, then marijuana, and on to cocaine or opiates.

***Treatment of Addiction by Neuro-Electric Acupuncture (NEAP).*** NEAP is an effective method for treating drug dependencies (19). The equipment used dispenses 2-100 hertz (cycles per second), electrical pulses given for periods of 20 to 30 minutes a day. Needles are not necessary, as the conducting polymer pads act as efficient conductors of the current.

In treatment, pad electrodes are placed over the classical Chinese *Hoku* points on the web between the thumb and first finger. This is actually the motor point of the dorsal interosseus muscle. This point is important because the thumb has the largest representation on the surface of the brain. Thus, a maximum number of brain cells are stimulated by this point.

A Dense/Disperse frequency setting producing an alternation of 2-100 hertz has been shown by analysis of cerebro-spinal fluid during stimulation to elevate Beta endorphin, met-enkephalins, dynorphins and ACTH at various locations in the brain, but particularly the arcuate nucleus of the hypothalamus and the anterior pituitary gland. This is the basis for its use in treating addiction.

## Recent Advances in the Use of Neuro-Electric Acupuncture

Although originally used for the treatment of pain and addiction, electro-acupuncture has been useful in other areas of medicine.

In a blinded, controlled study, electro-acupuncture given daily to hospitalized depressed patients was found to be as efficacious as a standard 200 mg daily dose of amitriptyline. Also, the patients receiving electro-acupuncture did not suffer the uncomfortable side effects seen with pharmacological treatment (20).

Several workers have noted that electro-acupuncture can be useful in the treatment of gastrointestinal disorders. It can induce homeostasis in an overactive colon and can effectively reduce gastric acidity (21,22).

Workers from Sweden reported that if electro-acupuncture is started within ten days of a stroke and continued on a daily basis, morbidity can be reduced and the time in nursing home care cut in half (23). In addition, there can be a normalization of postural control after a stroke (24).

Clinical studies have confirmed the specificity of stimulus frequency in electro-acupuncture treatments. A study from Sweden compared patients with low back pain receiving needles alone and needles with electrical stimulation at 2 hz and at 100 hz. Although the patients all showed some initial improvement, only those treated with electro-acupuncture at 2 hz had lasting relief (25). Stimulation at 100 hz, however, was found to be more effective than 2 hz for the treatment of spasticity resulting from spinal injuries (26).

Based on the observation that stimulation at 2 hz releases endorphins in the human CNS, we have applied the principle of conditioning in the treatment of patients with various psychiatric and psychosomatic conditions in which anxiety is a prominent feature (27). We have been encouraged to do this by reports that such release of neuropeptides can occur in animals using a bell as the conditional stimulus. More appropriate for our patients is the use of a meaningful mental image as the conditional stimulus. During stimulation that releases endorphins, we expose the patient to a relaxation tape encouraging the imaging of a familiar relaxing scene that will then become the conditional stimulus. At home, the patient is instructed to use this imaging technique several times a day. The purpose is to promote a means for the self-release of healing neuropeptides. This, then — a combination of a psychological stimulus and a physiological healing response — would be a clear example of "mind/body" medicine.

In conclusion, it seems evident that not only is electrical stimulation essential for the best clinical results with acupuncture, but that a developing body of evidence supports the assumption that specific frequencies will ultimately be indicated for specific types of problems. Thus, it is not the needles, points, or *meridians*, but rather the parameters of electrical stimulation that become the salient factors in treatment. As long as the electrodes, pads, or needles are placed in such a way as to promote the stimulation's ready access to the nervous system, i.e., motor points or points adjacent to major nerves, any reference to classical acupuncture points or *meridians* is unnecessary. Simply stated, NEAP is a method for getting a specific frequency of electrical stimulation into the central nervous system to promote the release of specific healing neurohumors.

## REFERENCES

1. Vieth, I. (1949). *The yellow emperor's classic of internal medicine.* Berkeley, CA: University California Press.
2. Ulett, G. (1992). *Beyond Yin and Yang: How acupuncture really works.* St. Louis, MO: Warren H. Green.
3. Liu, K.; Varela, M.; & Oswald, R. The correspondence between some motor points and acupuncture loci. *Amer J Chin Med, 3,* 347-358.
4. Gunn, C., (1978). Motor points and motor lines. *Amer J Acupuncture, 6,* 55-58.

5. Travell, J., & Simons, D. (1990). *Myofascial pain and dysfunction: The trigger point manual.* (Vols. 1 & 2). Baltimore, MD: Williams &Wilkins.
6. Melzack, R., & Wall, P. (1965). Pain mechanism: A new theory. *Science, 150,* 971-973.
7. Pert, C., & Snyder, S. (1973). Opiate receptors: Demonstration in nervous tissue. *Science, 179,* 1011-1014.
8. Kosterlitz, H., & Hughes, J. (1975). Some thoughts on the significance of enkephalin, the endogenous ligand. *Life Science, 19,* 91-96.
9. Mayer, D.; Price, D.; & Raffi, A. (1977). Antagonisim of acupuncture analgesia in man by the narcotic antagonist naloxone. *Brain Res, 121,* 368-372.
10. Sjolund, B.; Terenius, L.; & Erikesson, M. (1977). Increased cerebrospinal fluid levels of endorphins after electro-acupuncture. *Acta Physiol Scand, 100,* 382-384.
11. Peets, J., & Pomeranz, B. (1978). CXBX mice deficient in opiate receptors show poor electro-acupuncture analgesia. *Nature, 273,* 675-676.
12. Han, J.S., (1987). *The neurochemical basis of pain relief by acupunture. A collection of papers.* Beijing, China: Beijing Medical University.
13. Han, J.S., & Sun, S.L. (1990). Differential release of enkephalin and dynorphin by low and high frquency electro-acupuncture in the central nervous system. *Acupuncture, The Scientific International Journal, 1,* 19-27.
14. Nogier, P. (1972). *Treatise of auriculotherapy.* Moulins les Metz, France: Maisonneuve.
15. Melzack, R., & Katz, J. (1984). Auriculotherapy fails to relieve chronic pain. A controlled crossover study. *JAMA, 251,* 1041-1043.
16. Wen, H., & Cheung, S. (1973). Treatment of drug addiction by acupuncture and electrical stimulation. *Asian J Med, 9,* 138-141.
17. Lewith, C., & Machin, D. (1983). On the evaluation of the clinical effects of acupuncture. *Pain, 16,* 111-127.

18. Tyler, B.; Caldwell, C.; & Ghia, J. (1982). Transcutaneous electrical nerve stimulation: An alternative approach to the management of postoperative pain. *Anesth Analg, 61*, 449-56.
19. Ulett, G., & Nichols, J. (1995). *Handbook of N.E.A.P.* N.S.W. Australia: Novena Marketing.
20. Lou, H., et al. (1990). A comparative study of the treatment of depression by electro-acupuncture. *Acupuncture: The Scientific International Journal, 1*, 20-26.
21. Li, Y., et al. (1992). The effect of acupuncture on gastrointestinal function and disorders. *Amer J Gastroenterology, 87*, 1372-1381.
22. Jin, H., et al. (1992). The inhibition by electrical acupuncture on gastric acid secretion is mediated via endorphin and somatostatin in dogs. *Clin Res, 40*, 167A.
23. Johansson, K., et al. (1993). Can sensory stimulation improve the functional outcome in stroke patients? *Neurol, 43*, 2189-2192.
24. Magnusson M.; Johansson K.; & Johansson B. (1994). Sensory stimulation with electro-acupuncture promotes normalization of postural control after stroke. *Stroke: J Cerebr Circ, 25*, 1176-1180.
25. Thomas, M., & Lundberg, T. (1994). Importance of modes of acupuncture in the treatment of chronic nociceptive low back pain. *Acta Anesth Scand, 38*, 63-69.
26. Han, J.S., et al. (1994). Transcutaneous electrical nerve stimulation for treatment of spinal spasticity. *Chin Med J, 107*, 6-11.
27. Ulett, G. (1996). Conditioned healing with electro-acupuncture. *Alternative Therapies.* (In press).

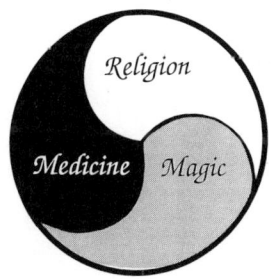

# XI

# CONCLUSION: A PRACTICAL APPROACH TO ALTERNATIVE MEDICINE

So WHAT HAVE WE LEARNED about alternative medicine? Where can its methods be of use in our health care system? Is there something of value for current allopathic medicine?

As for diagnosis, scientific allopathic medicine wins hands down. Admittedly, the longer, more detailed history-taking by the naturopath and homeopath creates better rapport with the patient. Particularly with chronic conditions, such careful attention to how the patient lives and thinks may assist in helping design a better life style. When serious illness is suspected, however, there is no alternative to modern laboratory diagnostic methods. When scientific diagnostic methods fail to reveal a recognized treatable illness and symptoms become chronic, people are likely to seek out an alternative therapist.

These days — when time is at a premium — pressured physicians often do not conduct the careful physical examinations that were performed in the days when the general practitioner had to rely on his senses of smell, sight, and palpation of the body to make the diagnosis. Today, the laboratory confirms the diagnosis speedily and with greater efficiency. X-rays and a host of non-invasive procedures quickly give a far more accurate diagnosis, taking but little of the physician's time. True, they cost more, but after all, you have only one life, and who can put a price on an accurate diagnosis when serious health problems must be promptly discovered if one's very existence hangs in the balance?

The spurious diagnostic methods of iridology, palmistry, astrology, pulse diagnosis, radiesthesia, diagnostic kinesiology, cranial-osteopathy, reflexology, Korean tongue diagnosis, O-Ring diagnosis, and a host of others should be avoided. These methods are not only worthless, but the delay occasioned by their use can be dangerous to one's health.

Turning to the treatment methods of alternative medicine, which of these can be helpful adjuncts in an overall health care system? We may summarize as follows:

1. The main benefit to be found in the major systems of alternative medicine can be spelled with a big "P" for Prevention. Emphasis on the whole person, mind, and body leads to an examination of habits of diet and exercise and a look at what is practiced in psychiatry — attention to the emotional side of life. It is not that allopathic medicine does not know this, but that under the pressure of today's busy practice, it is too often neglected. The new generation of physicians must be taught that an holistic approach can sometimes be as important as knowing the proper antibiotic for a specific infection.

2. The high cost of medical care today is largely generated by poor health habits. Sedentary life style, improper diets with too much fat and cholesterol, insufficient vitamin intake, and a failure to recognize the patient's idiosyncrasies, including food sensitivities, all play a role in disease prevention. Tobacco use alone was responsible for over 400,000 deaths last year. The abuse of alcohol added another 100,000. Even though the death rate from street drugs is only a few thousand fatalities each year, we have failed to properly address addiction as a medical and not a legal problem. The resulting "war on drugs" has produced an uncontrolled crime wave costing untold lives and dollars.

These are all matters that should be high on the list for the physician's attention. They are not "treatment" *per se*, but they are essential considerations in any long-range plan of health care for the nation. It would be interesting if our doctors were paid in the fashion once popular in China. At that time the doctor was paid only as long as the patient remained well. Payment stopped when the patient became ill!

3. Contrary to what one might think from loaded bookstore shelves and TV and radio commercials, there is no such thing as a "reducing diet." A sound diet yes, devoid of the *Yin/Yang* trappings or mysterious eating rituals. Many of the recommendations espoused by alternative medicine

can be simply stated as: "a primarily vegetarian diet eaten in moderate quantity with low fat, increased fiber, and adequate vitamins and minerals." For weight loss and good physical health, "at least 20 minutes a day of aerobic exercise" should be added.

4. The great variety of massage therapies with exotic oils, pressure points, breathing techniques, martial arts, and the like are OK if you like them. Better still is to enroll in an exercise program, *tai chi* or *yoga*, if you wish, but most importantly with other folks who will increase and support your own motivation. Once you are into any type of exercise program, the endorphin boost you get may be sufficient to keep you addicted to exercise.

5. Herbal preparations and supplemental vitamins and minerals may be fine if they are carefully monitored by knowledgeable persons. Be aware, however, that herbs are food, not medicines, and that too-large doses of vitamins or minerals can be toxic. Although homeopathic physicians may administer useful herbs, the basic principles of their practice are highly questionable. Dilutions that remove all of the original medicine, substances that resemble the organs to be treated, and drugs that accentuate symptoms of the illness — these practices lack scientific validation. When you are sick and the cause is known, it is best to take a specific approved medicine or herb that has been tested and shown to have a greater action than merely placebo. That is the safest way to go. Some carefully selected herbs, vitamins, and minerals, taken properly, may possibly increase the action of the body's immune system and thus might be good preventive measures.

6. When the body is in pain, joints are aching, or healing is not going well, various manipulative therapies such as chiropractic, osteopathy, biofeedback, neuroelectric acupuncture, or TENS may be helpful. Surely, such conservative treatments are worth a first try if they help avoid major surgical procedures which do not always bring complete relief. Harsher treatments can be reserved for use should conservative methods fail.

7. Increased knowledge of mind/body relationships and psychoimmunology point to the usefulness of various forms of alternative medicine that have existed because of their strong placebo value. If you

# Conclusion: A Practical Approach to Alternative Medicine

believe in a treatment and want to try it, just be sure it is not designed to lighten your wallet instead of your burden of discomfort. Studies point to the healing benefits of religious belief for those who have a strong commitment. Similar mechanisms appear to apply when there is a strong faith in the efficacy of some of the treatment methods of alternative medicine.

8. Finally, we have seen that there is no mysterious body energy. From the molecular and atomic make-up of the human body and from the healing effects seen with electrical stimulation of TENS units and neuro-electric acupuncture, there is reason to believe that in the future, new treatments may well result from investigations of electro-magnetic methods. There is little reason to believe that the electrons that may be floating about the surface of the hands of self-proclaimed "healers" have as much effect as the demonstrated currents of neuro-electric acupuncture.

In conclusion, some effects of alternative medicine appear to be not just magic or mystery. Some may have underlying biochemical and neurophysiological mechanisms that are effective beyond placebo. Those treatments appearing to have some surface validity may be candidates for further careful scientific exploration. They might stand the test of double-blind evaluation. Traditional Chinese acupuncture became "scientized" to yield the useful and factually proven technique of neuro-electric acupuncture. Others in the portfolio of holistic healers could follow the same path and become part of accepted medical practice.

Our health care delivery system seems to be moving in the direction of primary care. Proven alternative methods fit well into the tool kit of the family practitioner whose orientation is strongly preventive. Perhaps here, Eastern and Western concepts can be integrated into a medical practice that will thus become more adjunctive than alternative.

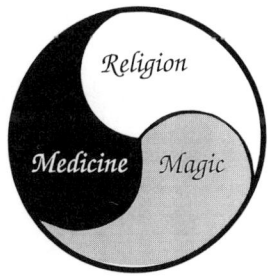

# Selecting a Good Doctor of Alternative Medicine

License and diploma current and prominently displayed.

Member of state society.

Member of national organizations.

Sloppy clinic — careless doctor.

Avoid "New Age" clinics. *Chakras*, energy, *ch'i*, *meridian* pathways, past life experiences, rebirthing, crystals, and flower therapy are signals for caution. Such "doctors" are not likely to know what is best for you.

Avoid clinics that treat everyone the same way, i.e., "hypnotists" and "acupuncturists." Different diseases and different patients require different therapies.

Beware the "assembly line" office or doctors who spend little time with you.

Avoid doctors who use unusual diagnostic procedures, test your muscles or hair, and then sell you their own brand of vitamins or herbals.

Finally, if it looks "goofy," it probably is goofy.

# NAME INDEX

## A
Achterberg, J., 78
Akil, H., 59
Akpinar, S., 95
Albert, L., 58
Alexander, F. Matthias, 143
Allen, G., 77
Amsterdam, E., 57
Andresen, G., 97
Argyle, M., 72, 77
Atherton, D., 19
Atkin, 184
Avicenna, 156

## B
Bach, Edward, 142
Backman, H., 57
Baldwin, H., 57
Barber, T. X., 95
Barlow, W., 153
Barnum, P.T., xvii, 100
Barrett, S., 112, 115, 191, 192
Beatty, J., 95
Becker, P., 96
Becker, R., 9, 18
Beecher, H.K., 52, 53, 54, 56, 74, 78
Beecher, J., 57
Beit-Hallaham, B., 72, 77
Benson, Herbert T., 17, 19, 57, 80, 94
Berger, 184
Bergson, Henri, 8, 39
Bernard, Claude, xiv, 9, 19, 79, 94
Bernheim, Hippolyte, 88
Berry, T., 113, 115
Bertrand, Alexander, 87
Beyerstein, B., 86, 95

Bickel, W., 49, 115
Bierre, P., 91, 93, 96
Biggs, S.J., 137
Binkert, E., 55, 58
Blackburn, G., 191
Blackmore, S., 48
Blackstone, Harry, Sr., 23
Blackstone, Harry, Junior, 23
Blumberg, D., 47, 114
Booth, J., 48
Bosch, Hieronymus, 22
Bounemeaux, H., 57
Braid, James, 87, 88
Brenman, 89
Breuer, Joseph, 88
Briggs, A., 57
Brody, H., 58
Brook, R., 129, 153
Brown, A., 96
Brown, Barbara, 84, 95
Brown, D., 48
Brown, E., 48
Brown, M., 153
Brown, N., 192
Brown, R., 175
Bruegel, Pieter the Elder, 22
Burr, H.S., 9, 18
Burrow, J., 175
Butler, Kurt, 120, 152, 175
Byrd, R., 76

## C
Caldwell, C., 217
Cannon, Walter, 10, 19, 79, 94
Carter, M., 114
Carver, William, 130
Cayce, Edgar, 27, 28, 35, 106

Cham, 22
Charcot, Jean Martin, 88, 89
Che, P.H., 6, 18, 77
Cheung, S., 216
Chiribin, J., 68, 77
Chretien, M., 58
Christopher, M., 48
Cleghorn, R., 59
Cobb, Stanley, 10, 19
Comstock, G., 71, 77
Coon, D., 48
Copperfield, David, 23
Coue, Emile, 88
Cranston, Leroy, 30
Cranston, Margie, 30
Crawford, H., 44, 49, 90, 91, 96
Culpepper, Nicholas, 158
Culver, R., 48, 115
Cushing, Harvey, 132

**D**

Daumier, 22
Davis, W., 47
de Puysequr, Marquis, 87
Descartes, xv, 44
de Vernejoul, Pierre, 197
Devloo, R., 57
DeWied, D., 59
Dionne, R., 58
Dioscorides, 155
Dixon, Jeanne, 35
Dossey, Larry, 65, 66, 76, 100, 114
Downing, G., 153
Dowson, S., 57
Doyle, Conan, 30
Dunninger, J., 48

**E**

Eddy, Mary A. Morse Glover Patterson, 66

Einstein, Albert, 31, 46, 65
Eisenberg, D., xiii, xviii
Elliotson, John, 87, 89
Ellis, Albert, 70
Ellis, J., 192
En-lai, Chou, 103
Enroth, R., 77
Erickson, 89
Erikesson, M., 203, 216
Esdaile, James, 87
Evans, W., 57

**F**

Faria, Abbe, 87
Feldenkrais, Moshe, 143, 153
Fields, H., 58
Fisher, P., 19
Fisher-Rizzi, S., 153
Frank, A., 183, 191
Freud, Sigmund, 70, 88, 146
Fromm, Erich, 96

**G**

Gaby, A., 181
Gach, M., 154
Galen, 39, 155, 156
Galvani, xv
Gamez, A., 48
Gardner, Martin, 32, 48, 152
Gartner, 71, 72
Gassner, Father, 65
Geller, Uri, 33
Ghia, J., 217
Giles, C., 48
Gill, 89
Goodhart, George, 111, 115, 145, 154
Goldring, S., 19
Goldstein, A., 58

Index 225

Gordon, N., 58
Gorlin, R., 57
Graham, James, 66
Gravenstein, J., 57
Greatrakes, Valantine, 65
Green, Alyce, 49, 83, 95
Green, Elmer, 41, 49, 83, 95
Grenfell, R., 57
Grevert, P., 58
Grey, W., 48
Gringer, 89
Guadagno, C., 1 53
Gruzelier, J., 49, 96
Guillemin, R., 59
Guinness, A., 152
Gunn, C.C., 8, 18, 153, 203, 215
Gur, R., 95

## H

Haanen, H., 96
Hadfield, J.A., 89
Hahnemann, 170, 173
Haley, J., 96
Hall, G. Stanley, 31, 32
Han, J. Sheng, 8, 47, 203, 204, 216, 217
Han, Kim Bong, 197
Hargreaves, K., 58
Harrison, Tinsley, xvi
Heller, Joseph, 144, 153
Henkin, W., 153
Henning, Douglas, 23
Henry, W., 69, 77
Herbert, V., 192
Hess, Walter, 10, 19
Hilgard, E., 44, 49, 90, 95, 96
Hilgard, J., 44, 49, 96
Hippocrates, 104, 155, 156, 170
Hoffer, Abram, 191, 192

Hohenlohe, Prince von, 65
Holland, W., 57
Hollister, L., 57
Hopson, J., 19
Horsley, 89
Houdin, Robert, 22, 47
Houdini, Harry, 23, 30 (*see also* Eric Weiss)
Hoyle, C., 57
Huard, P., 152
Hubbard, Ron, xvii
Hughes, J., 203, 216
Hull, B., 48
Hull, Clark, 69, 88
Hung, Ko, 128
Hyman, R., 115

## I

Ianna, P., 48, 115
Itil, T., 95

## J

Jacobs, Joseph, xiii, 100
Jacobsen, Edmond, 80, 92, 94, 96
James, William, 31
Janet, Pierre, 88
Jarvik, Murray, 56, 59
Jastrow, Joseph, 31
Jensen, Bernard, 109, 115
Jin, H., 217
Johansson, B., 217
Johansson, K., 217
Johnson, L., 85, 86, 95
Jolles, J., 59
Jones, Jim, 67

## K

Kaada, B., 58
Kalliola, H., 57

Kamiya, Joseph, 83, 94
Kane, B., 48
Katz, J., 216
Kaye, J., 96
Kimmey, M., 153
King, Zoser, 61
Kleinjen, J., 114, 170, 175
Kleitman, N., 49
Knipschild, P., 114, 115
Ko, S.M., 6, 18, 77
Kosterlitz, H.W., 59, 203, 216
Kriegel, M., 153
Krieger, Delores, 38, 144, 154
Kroger, W., 93, 96
Kua, E.H., 6, 18, 77
Kulkosky, P., 86, 95
Kunz, B., 154
Kunz, K., 154
Kurtz, P., 18, 49
Kushi, Michio, 185

## L

Larson, D., 6, 18, 69, 70, 71, 72, 77
Larson, S., 6, 18, 70, 71, 72, 77
Lasagna, L., 55, 56, 76, 78
Leao, A., 9, 19
Legewie, H., 95
Levin, J., 73, 77
Levine, K., 55, 58
Lewith, C., 211, 216
Lewith, G., 57
Li, Y., 18, 217
Liebeault, A.A., 87, 88
Liljequist, N., 109
Liu, K., 153, 203, 215
Liu, Y.H., 8, 18
Loh, Y., 58

Longstreth, G., 57
Loriaux, L., 58
Lou, H., 217
Lundberg, T., 217
Luthe, W., 94, 96

## M

Jachin, D., 57, 216
Mackowiak, P., 19
Magnusson, M., 217
Makhlouf, Charbel, 67
Malone, M., 96
Mao, Chairman, 7, 103, 206
Maslow, Abraham, 7
Mayer, D., 203, 216
McCallie, D., 57
McCann, L., 48
McCutcheon, L., 153
McGary, W.I., 114
Melanthcon, 69
Melzack, R., 86, 95, 203, 216
Mesmer, Franz Anton, 38, 66, 87, 89, 91
Mihic, D., 55, 58
Millay, J., 4, 8
Minagawa, R., 97
Mitas, J., 115
Moon, C., 96
Moyer, Bill, 40
Mueller, G., 58
Munro, xv, 39
Munsterberg, 32
Murray, M., 148, 181

## N

Nash, 96
Neame, A., 78
Nichols, J., 217

Nieuwenhuys, R., 58
Nogier, P., 206, 216
Nordenstrom, B., 9, 19
Nostradamus, 34
Nung, Emperor Shen, 11

## O

Ohsawa, George, 185
Omura, Yoshoki, 18, 111, 115
Orne, M., 95
Ornish, Dean, 185
Osler, Sir William, xiv
Osmond, Humphrey, 191, 192
Ostling, G., 57
Oswald, R., 18, 203, 215

## P

Palmer, B.J., 130
Palmer, Daniel David, 129
Palmer, D.D., 130, 131
Paracelsus, 156, 157
Partridge, K., 71, 77
Parwatikar, S., 18
Passarelli, E., 57
Pasteur, Louis, vii
Patterson, D., 96
Pauling, Linus, 191, 192
Peets, 203, 216
Peezely, Ignatz von, 109
Penfield, Wilder, 45, 49
Peniston, E., 86, 95
Perkins, Elisha, 99
Pert, Candice, 45, 47, 49, 203, 216
Peterson, D., 95
Pfeiffer, C., 192
Pinsky, R., 53, 58
Pomeranz, Bruce, 203, 209, 216
Porkert, M., 115, 123, 152
Pratkanis, A., 100, 114

Pratt, J.G., 32
Price, D., 216
Prince, Morton, 88
Puysegar, 89

## Q

Quimby, Pineas Parkhurst, 66

## R

Raffi, A., 216
Raso, Jack, 140, 153
Rawcliffe, D., 48
Reed, W., 97
Reich, Wilhelm, 146, 147, 154
Rhazes, 156
Rhine, J.B., 32
Rinzler, S., 59
Rolf, Ida, 143, 153
Romano, C., 22, 47
Rootenberg, J., 91, 93, 96
Rose, Louis, 62, 76
Roy, 23
Rush, Benjamin, 70

## S

Sabbagh, K., 99, 114
Sabourin, M., 90, 96
Sadd, S., 77
Sagan, Carl, 21, 47
Sanders, Mark, 136
Sarbin, T., 95
Schiller, P., 73, 77
Schmitt, W., 115
Schneider, N., 59
Schultz, Johannes, 80, 92, 94, 96
Schwartz, A., 162, 175
Schwartz, M., 95
Schweitzer, Albert, xiv
Seidman, M., 154

Seigel, B., xviii
Selye, Hans, 10, 19, 80, 94
Shapiro, A., 57
Shekelle, P., 129, 153
Sidis, Boris, 88
Siegel, Bernie, 76, 77
Sigfried, 23
Simes, Tollak B., 58
Simon, A., 115
Simons, D., 216
Simonton, O.C., 76, 78
Sims, H., 69, 77
Sjolund, B., 203, 216
Skolnick, Andrew, 104, 114, 152
Snyder, S., 49, 203, 216
Spiegel, David, 73, 77, 89, 91, 93, 96
Spiegel, H., 91, 93, 96
Spray, S., 69, 77
Stainberg, J., 96
Stearn, J., 47
Stern, J., 153
Still, Andrew Taylor, 137, 138
Stone, Randolph, 144
Strohecker, J., 115, 152, 175
Strube, M., 96
Stunkard, Albert, 182, 191
Sullivan, M., 175
Sun, S.L., 216
Swaab, D., 58
Sydenham, Thomas, xv
Szara, S., 58

## T
Tansley, D., 115
Tart, C., 94
Tavris, C., 72, 77
Terenius, L., 203, 216
Ter Reit, G., 114
Thomas, M., 217
Thomas, R., 95
Thurston, 23
Tollison, C., 153
Trager, Milton, 144, 153
Traut, E., 57
Travell, J., 216
Turner, William, 157
Tyler, B., 217
Tyler, V., 181

## U
Ulett, George A., ix, 18, 95, 115, 153, 215, 217
Ullman, M., 49, 95
Upledger, J., 154
Usui, Mikao, 145

## V
Vanderpool, H., 73, 77
Varela, M., 18, 203, 215
Vieth, I., 215
Vogt, E., 115
von Ulm, 22

## W
Wadden, T., 191
Wall, P., 86, 95, 203, 216
Ward, A., 19
Watkins, A., 49, 115
Wayne, E., 57
Wedding, D., 58
Weiss, Eric, 22
Wen, H., 208, 216
Willett, W., 192
Williams, Roger, 191, 192
Wilson, D., 71, 77

Index 229

Withering, William, 12, 158
Witmer, J., 77
Wolberg, Lewis, 89
Wolf, S., 53, 58
Wolfson, S., 57
Wolk, S., 56
Wolman, B., 49, 95
Wong, M., 152
Worthen, D., 115
Wright, J., 181

Wright, P., 28, 48
Wu, Xianghong, 38, 49

**Y**
Yates, A., 58
Yogi, Maharishi Mahesh, 120
Young, H., 99, 114

**Z**
Zarathustra, 61
Zimmerman, M., 77

# SUBJECT INDEX

**A**
Absent prayer, 65
  use by radio and television healers, 67
Acupuncture, 3, 196-215
  acupuncture points, 123
  addiction and, 213-214
  ancient, 197-202
  by chiropractors, 132
  *ch'i*, 39, 40, 122, 127, 197-198 (*see also* Body energies)
  comparison hypnosis and, 203
  conditions responding to, 196
  culture and politics involvement in, 103-104
  ear acupuncture, 206
  "gate theory," 203
  *hsueh*, acupuncture points, 123, 197, 198
  in U.S., 202
  main purpose of, 8
  *meridians* theory, 8, 103, 108, 122, 197, 199, 201
    traditional, table, 198
    unpaired, table, 198
  moxabustion defined, 201
  neuro-electric, 202-208 (*see also* Neuro-electric acupuncture)
  pain, 208-212 (*see also* Pain)
  points used, 8
  results research of, 7-8
  scientized, 11
  sinarteriology defined, 122, 197
  spread of use over centuries, 202
  technique of, 198
    *chun*, illustrated, 199
  use of, 144
Addiction, 213-214
  definition, 213
  features of, 213
  treatment of using neuro-electric acupuncture (NEAP), 213
    technique used, 213

types drugs leading to, 213
Alcohol abuse, role of "higher power" in recovery, 71
African witch doctor, success of, xiv
Alexander massage technique, 143
Allopathic medicine
    best diagnostic methods, 218
    definition, 3
    doctrine of specific etiology, 159
    germ theory, 159
    Random Clinical Trial use in, 52
    treatment of, 148-152
        anxiety-insomnia, 148
        arthritis, 148
        asthma-hay fever, 149
        common cold, 150
        diabetes, 150
        headache, 151
        hypertension, 149
        peptic ulcer, 152
        prostate enlargement, 151
Alternative medicine
    alternative health defined, 140
    as response to consumer need, xvi-xvii
    basic approach to, viii-ix
    basis of, 6
    benefit of, viii
    conclusion, 218-222
    contributions to conventional medicine, 15-16
    definition, 3
    diagnostic methods of, 218-219
    emphasis on consumer participation, xiii
    evaluation by scientific investigation, xiv
    herbology, 11-13 (*see also* Herbology)
    incidence use by Americans, xiii
    life force and homeostasis, 8-10
    magic and mystery, 20-47 (*see also* Magic and mystery)
    magicians of, 23, 24 (*see also* Magic)
    methods of, 140-152
        aromatherapy, 141-142
        Bach Flower remedies, 142-143
        bodywork, 143-147 (*see also* Bodywork)
    movement toward advanced techniques, xvii
    need knowledge of Eastern medicine, 17
    of East and West, 3-18
        acupuncture (*see* Acupuncture)
        magical healing (*see* Shamanism)
        religious healings, 5
        similarities of, 4
        voodoo of Africa, 4
    prevention, 219
    preventive health team members, ix
    problems associated with, 7
    Reiki healing, 38
    Rosecrucian healing, 38
    roots of, 3-18
    selection, good doctor, of, table, 222
    sideshows of, 140-147
    techniques evaluated by FDA, 46
    Therapeutic Touch, 38

treatment methods of, summary, 219-221
treatment illness using
  anxiety-insomnia, 148
  arthritis, 148
  asthma-hay fever, 149
  common cold, 150
  diabetes, 150
  headache, 151
  hypertension, 149
  peptic ulcer, 152
  prostate enlargement, 151
use of placebos, 54
American Indians
  Navajo Indian healing by, 26
  power of the Great Spirit in healing, 40
  use of shaman, 25-26
American Society for Psychical Research, founding of, 31
Anxiety-insomnia
  allopathic treatment, 148
  alternative treatment, 148
Apoptosis, definition, 43
Aromatherapy, 141-142
  examples and uses of, 141-142
  placebo effect of, 141
  response emotions to, 141
  technique used, 141
Arthritis
  allopathic treatment, 148
  alternative treatment, 148
Asthma
  allopathic treatment, 149
  alternative treatment, 149
Astral projections, 32
Astrology
  astronomy versus, 35, 36
  belief in and metallic elements, 158
  origin of, 64
  preoccupation with today, 36
  unscientific methods of diagnosis involving, 106-107
Atkin's diet, 184
Autogenic training for relaxation, 80
Ayurvedic medicine, 116-121
  as pseudo medicine, 104
  body energy and, 117 (*see also* Body Energies)
  breath, prana, as, 40
  cause of illness and role physician, 118
  characteristics of body types, table, 118
  classification of all persons, 117
  curative practice, 119
  development of, xiv, xvii, 8
  emphasis of, 116
  meaning of term, 116
  oldest medical practice used, 116
  physician examination of patient in, 110
  *prana* defined, 39 (*see also* Body energies)
  preventive medicine, 119, 120
  regional differences in, 119
  treatments of, 116, 117, 120
  unscientific diagnostic methods, 110
  use relaxation in, 79 (*see also* Relaxation)
  *yoga* associated with, 17, 119 (*see also Yoga*)

## B

Bach Flower Remedies, 142-143
   preparation of, 142-143
   theory of, 142
Belief, definition, 21
Berger's immune power diet, 184-185
Beverly Hills Diet, 185
Biofeedback, 81-86
   definition, 81-82
   development of, 82
   effects techniques used, 82
   electrodermal, 84
   electroencephalographic, 83, 85-86
   electromyographic, 83-84
   feedback, 81
   somatic, 84
   thermal, 83
Bircher-Benner System Diet, 185
Body electro-acupuncture, 211
   (*see* Electro-acupuncture)
Body energies, 39-45
   auras, 40
   balance of *Yin* and *Yang*, 40-41
   biological energies, 42-43
   breathing as, 40
   cosmic origin of, 40-41
   external application of, 47
   function of nervous system, 161
      healing using, 46-47
   hydraulic theory, 39
   influence mind over, 45-46
   life energy, 45
   nervous energy, 43-45
   *Qi Gong* energy, 40
   quantum physics, 41-42
   power of God and religious healing, 39
   power of the Great Spirit in healing, 40
   presence of, 46
   "seat of the soul," 44
   sleep, 44
      stages of, 44
   subconscious, 45
   summary, 221
   Therapeutic Touch, 41-42
   thoughts, 45
   "travel from ear" theory of auriculotherapists, 40
   "travel from soles of feet" theory of reflexologists, 40
Bodywork
   therapeutic massage, 143-144
   use of term, 143

## C

Cancer and diet, 186-188
   animal fat and colon cancer, 187
   plants recommended for diet, 187
   possible role dietary fat in, 186-187
   recommendations diet intake, 187
   vitamin augmentation advised, 187-188
Chinese *meridians* (*see Meridians*)
Chiropractic medicine, 37-38, 128-137
   acceptance of, 136-137
      by allopathic physicians, 133
   accomplishments of, 136
   basic theory of, 130, 132
   criticisms of, 136

Index 233

debate regarding duties and responsibilities of, 129
definition, 131-132
exclusion from Medicare Act, 132
founding of, 37-38
history of, 129-131
  founder of, 129
  original doctrine of, 130-131, 132
  school to train doctors, 130
incidence back problems, 128-129
lack regulatory body for, 130
malpractice and, 133
meaning of term, 128
methods of diagnosis and treatment, 134-136
  classes of adjustments, 134
  diagnostic experimental instruments, 135
  drugless pain-control techniques, 135
  extent of physical examination, 134
  high velocity, low amplitude adjusting (HVLA), 134
  low force adjusting, 134-135
  nerve stimulation techniques, 136
  preventive care, 135
  soft tissue techniques, 135
number licensed today, 131
origin of term, 129

philosophy of, 131-132
referrals for treatment of medical conditions, 137
spinal manipulation for low back pain, 137
subluxation complex
  definition, 133
  etiology of, 133-134
  founder's concept, 129, 130, 132
  training for today, 131
  schism existing, 131
  treatment methods added to, 132
Christian Science
  description of, 67
  founding of, 66-67
  healings testified to, 75
CISCOP, *Qi Gong* energy studied by, 4-5, 40
Clairvoyance, 31
Clinical acupuncture (*see* Electro-acupuncture)
Color puncture, 146
Committee for the Scientific Investigation of Claims of the Paranormal (CISCOP), 4-5
Common cold
  allopathic treatment, 150
  alternative treatment, 150
Complementary medicine (*see also* Alternate medicine)
  provision for in Europe, 16-17
Conventional medicine
  basis of, 6
  contributions of to alternative medicine, 15-16
  definition, 3
  impediments to evaluation

treatment efficacy, 13-15
  placebo effect, 14, 15
  research methods, 14
  role of WHO, 13
 problems of, 6-7
 treatment in, 6
Cranio-sacral therapy, 145

**D**

Dean Ornish's diet, 185
Depression, effect religious commitment on, 72
Designer drugs, 1 67- 1 68
 cardiac drugs, 168
 to treat depression and manic depression, 167-168
 to treat schizophrenia, 168
Diabetes
 allopathic treatment, 150
 alternative treatment, 150
Diet and vitamins, 182-191
 cancer and diet, 186-188
 dietary reconsideration, table, 188
 obesity problem, 182-186 (*see also* Obesity)
  vitamins and minerals, 189-191
Divination, 34-36
 astrology, 35-36
 from Old Testament, 34
 milfoil lots methods, 35
 precognition, 31, 34
 predictions of Nostradamus, 34
 scapulomancy, method of, 35
 Tarot method, 35
 uses of, 35
Divorce and marital satisfaction, role church attendance in, 72

Doctor, derivation of word, xvi
Dowsing, 113, 114
 sex detector machine, 114
Drug, source of term, 160
Drug abuse, relation to absence of religion in life, 71-72

**E**

Ear acupuncture
 basis of, 206-207
 diagram of, 206
 innervation of, diagram, 207
 uses of, 208
Eastern medicine
 acupuncture (*see* Acupuncture)
 conclusion, 16-18
 herbology (*see* Herbology)
 impediment to acceptance in West, 17
 integration Western and, 16, 17
 knowledge modern technique needed, 17
 lack acceptance techniques in West, 17
  scientization techniques, 17
 life force and homeostasis, 8-10
 medical paradigms, 15-16
 placebo effect, 14, 15 (*see also* Placebo effect)
 religious healing, 5-6
 scientizing Traditional Chinese Medicine, 7-8, 17
  examples, 17
 shamanism (*see* Shamanism)
 Traditional Chinese Medicine (*see* Traditional Chinese Medicine)
Electro-acupuncture (*see also* Neuro-electric acupuncture)

technique of, 211
   electrical stimulation, 212
   frequency of treatments, 212
   insertion needles, diagram, 212
   length time of each treatment, 212
   use for pain control, 211-212
   results obtained, 211
   voltage used for, 41
Electrodermal biofeedback, 84
Electroencephalographic biofeedback, 85-86
Electromyographic biofeedback, 83-84
Energy medicine, 146
Extrasensory perception (ESP), definition, 31-32

## F

Faith, definition, 21, 74
Faith healing, 60-76
   continuing power of shrines, 74-75
   effect religious commitment
      alcohol abuse, 71
      depression, 72
      divorce and marital satisfaction, 72
      drug abuse, 71-72
      general well being, 72
      juvenile delinquency, 72
      physical health, 72-73
      suicide, 71
   exploiters of, 23
   focus of on body, mind, and soul, 68
   healing by royalty members, 64
   historical, 61-67

   absent prayer, 65
   after death of healer, 67
   astrology and, 64
   belief illness God's preordained punishment, 64
   by churches of all major religions, 64
      by Jesus of Nazareth, 62
      by television and radio personalities, 67
      early references to healing, 61
      first recorded physician, 61
      healing by hypnosis, 66
      healing practices, 64
      healing without religious creeds, 64-65
      inability to document, 62
      Jewish Hasidic Movement, 66
      lack proven cures, 67
      mind/body medicine, 65-66
      polytheistic ancient religions, 61
      potential financial profit of, 67
      pragmatic healers, 64-65
      prayer brings divine intervention and cure, 61-62
      prior to this century, 60
   holistic medicine (*see* Holistic

medicine)
importance brain peptides, 76
involvement CNS and immune system in, 75-76
modern healing, 68-70
  attitude psychiatry toward religion, 69-70
  attitudes toward Jesus, 68-69
  emphasis on cause of disease, 68
  of most faiths, 68
  percent patients with self-limiting disorders, 68
  percent psychiatrists religious, 69
  reemphasis on total person, 68
  use petitional prayers to God, 68
possible physiological basis of health producing phenomenon, 74-76
  attitude of care given, 74
  belief in power of prayer, 75
  conclusions, 75-76
  placebo response, 74
role imagery in, 76
specific areas of study, 71-74
studies religion and health, 70-74
  extrinsic religious commitment, 70-71
  intrinsic religious commitment, 70
  types of prayers, 70
  use of confession, 71
use of term, 62
Feldenkrais massage method, 143

Folk medicine, 11 (*see also* Herbology)
  in China, 11
  in Europe, 11-12

## H

Hair analysis in diagnosis, 112
Hasidic faith healing, 66
Hay Diet, 185
Headache
  allopathic treatment, 151
  alternative treatment, 151
Healing
  by faith (*see* Faith healing)
  techniques that help body heal, 60
Hellerwork massage technique, 144
Herbology, 11-13
  homeopathy and (*see* Herbology and homeopathy)
  origin of, 155
  pharmacopeia in year 1000 A.D., 51
  practice of in Japan, 12
  results recent conference on, 12-13
  use of term, 12
  use Traditional Chinese Medicine, 11
Herbology and homeopathy, 155-181
  advances in purification of, 159
  AMA Council on Pharmacy and Chemistry, 166
  astrology and, 158
  attitude German medical schools toward, 166
  classification as foodstuffs, 165
  comparison prescription drug

and herbal preparations
  costs development, 165
  profits from, 165
  sales promotion, 166
  regulations for, 166
definition, 155
doctrine of signatures, 158
earliest records of use, 155
father of pharmaceutical
  chemistry, 156-157
financial costs of, 165
first herbal industry by Shakers,
  158-159
for purging, 158
"germ theory," 159
green wave of interest in, 164
human physiology dictator of
  action of drugs, 160-164
    action herb on cell receptor, 161
    body energy, 151
    cells of systems of body,
      160-161
    delay in obtaining FDA
      approval drugs, 162
    determination site and
      manner drugs act,
      161-162
    function of nervous system,
      161
    patents for drugs, 162-163
    purification crude plant
      materials, 162
    regulation drug dosage,
      162-163
  side effects of drugs, 163
  side effects of herbs, 163-164
modern pharmaceuticals, 167-170
  development designer
    drugs, 167-168
  toxic side effects of herbs,
    169-170
monastic medicine, 156
natural remedies, 166-167
  table, 177
packaging of, 167
preparation infusions, teas,
  decoctions, 167
primitive drug and modern
  derivative, table, 176
publications of preparations of,
  158
questionable "cure-all" nature
  herbal formulas, 164
recording knowledge of, 156
salves against supernatural
  creatures, 156
shelf life of, 167
study British flora, 157
summary, 220
toxicity some herbs, 165
used in prescriptions, 165
  table, 176
use in U.S., 158
use of bleeding, 156
use term "Certified Organically
  Grown," 167
use term phytotherapy or
  botanical medicine in
    Europe, 166
variations in medicinal properties of, 160
widely used herbal preparations, 169
  table, 177-181
work with metals purification,
  156-157
Hippocrates era, illness and four

humors, xiv, 156
Holistic, use of term, xiii-xiv
Holistic medicine, use relaxation in, 79
Holistic healing medicine
   healers belief theirs is the only, 46
   introduction concepts of, 68
   placebo effect in, 52
Holistic hokum and doubtful diagnosis, 98-114
   desirable and doubtful diagnostic procedures, 104-114
      accurate diagnosis needed, 104-105
      basis of, 105
      fringe medicine as alternative, 99
      laboratory procedures needed, 105
      unscientific methods of diagnosis, 106-116
   mechanical tractor of 1797, 99
   nutritional myth, 99
   quackery, 98
      unicorn horn use, 98
   selling pseudomedicine, 99-104
   unscientific methods of diagnosis, 106-114
      astrological diagnosis, 106-107
      Ayurvedic medicine (*see* Ayurvedic medicine)
      hair analysis, 112
      homeopathy, 110-111
      iridology, 109
      kinesiology and O-Ring diagnostics, 111-112
      palmistry, 112-113
      psionic diagnosis, 113-114
      radioesthesia, 113
      radionics, 113
      Shamanic diagnosis, 106
      Traditional Chinese Medicine, 108-110
Homeopathy
   basis of, 12
   by chiropractors, 132
   greatest asset of, 173
   growth of, 170-171
   homeopathy and herbs (*see also* Herbology and homeopathy)
   impact during Asiatic cholera epidemic of 1832, 170-171
   "like cures like" theory, 170
   major principals of, 171-172
      Law of Infinitesimals, 171, 172
      law of similars, 170, 171-172
      miasma, 171, 172
      potentization, 171, 172
      provings, 170, 172
      trituration and succussion, 171, 172
   principles of by Hippocrates, 170
   treatment, 6
   unscientific diagnosis of, 110-111
   use body's natural healing processes, 173
Homeostasis
   contributions to understanding of, 9-10
   definition, 10
   use of term, 79

# Index

Ho'opono Pono, 146
Hydraulic theory, xv, 39
Hypertension
    allopathic treatment, 149
    alternative treatment, 149
Hypnosis
    animal magnetism of Mesmer, 38
    as technique, not treatment, 66, 94
    biological versus environmental responses, 91-92
    clinical situation uses of, 38, 66, 91
    definition, 89
    early leaders in field, 87-89
    EEG research results, 90-91
    factors in success of, 90
    founder of, 38
    history of use, 87
    hypnoanalysis, 89
    induction techniques, 92
    nature of, 89-92
    publication journals related to, 89
    stages of by Charcot, 88
    study trance state, 89-90
    use relaxation, 79 (*see also* Relaxation)
    uses of, 38, 92-94
        control nosebleeds, 93
        control of pain, 92-93
        cure warts, 93
        in childbirth, 93
        in field of psychiatry, 93-94
        side effects chemotherapy, 93
        stage entertainment, 93

## I

*I Ching*, 4
Iridology
    by chiropractors, 132
    diagnosis by, 109-110
        use colored photographs today, 109
    double-blind studies results, 110

## J

Jogger's high, 210
Juvenile delinquency
    religious participation as deterrent to, 72

## K

Karuna reiki, 146
Kinesiology
    applied use of, 145
    diagnostics, 111-112
    purpose invention of, 111

## L

Laserpuncture, 146
Laying on of hands healing, 37-38
    (*see also* Mystical healing)
Life force (*see* Body energies)
Life force and homeostasis, 8-10
    characteristics necessary to living organism, 9
    contributions to understanding of, 9-10
    definition life force, 9

## M

Macrobiotics, 185
Magic and mystery, 20-47
    astrology and, 21

body energies, 39-45 (*see also* Body energies)
by Houdini, 22-23
conclusion, 45-47
divination, 34-36 (*see also* Divination)
faith healing, 23
magicians and illusionists today, 23
mystical healing, 37-38 (*see also* Mystical healing)
parapsychology, 31-33 (*see also* Parapsychology)
preventative medicine stressed by, 24
*Qi Gong* (*see Qi Gong*)
relationship to religion and healing, 20
Shamanism, 24-28 (*see also* Shamanism)
spiritualism, 29-31 (*see also* Spiritualism)
types of in healing, 21-22
use in Middle Ages, 22
use to influence primitive people, 22
Magical healing (*see* Shamanism)
*Mansin*, Korean, 4
Massage, therapeutic, 143-145
    acupressure (*see* Acupressure)
    Alexander technique, 143
    Feldenkrais method, 143
    Hellerwork technique, 144
    Polarity therapy, 144
    Reflexology, 144
    Rolfing massage, 143-144
    Therapeutic Touch, 144-145
    Trager approach, 144
Medicine
    alternative (*see* Alternative medicine)
    as scientific, xvi
    belief illness due four humors, xiv
    chiropractic, 37-38
    complementary, 16-17
    conventional (*see* Conventional medicine)
    during Middle Ages, xv
    Eastern (*see* Eastern medicine)
    focus on patient as a person, xvii
    germ theory during 17th Century, xv
    homeopathic versus allopathic physicians, xvi
    mind/body interaction, xvii
    New Age, 46
    progress past century, vii
    progress through 19th Century, xv
*Meridians*
    in Traditional Chinese Medicine, 8, 103, 108, 122
    lack proof existence of, 122-123
    number of, 123
Mystical healing, 37-38
    by hypnosis, 37
    chiropractic medicine, 37-38
    definition, 37
    hypnosis, 38
    of Biblical times, 37
    *Qi Gong* (*see Qi Gong*)
    techniques of, 38

# N

Navajo Indian medicine man, 25-27
    healing by, 27
        ceremonies of, 25-26

selection of, 26
use of herbology, 26
Naturopathy, 173-175
　definition, 175
　degree for, 174
　　studies for, 174
　description of, 174
　homeopathy and, 173
　licenses for, 174
　principles of, 173-174, 175
　purpose of, 173
Near death experiences (NDE), 32
Neuro-electric acupuncture, 202-208, 214-215
　decreased pain using, 210
　development of, 204-205
　recent advances in use of, 214-215
　results studies of, 205
　　graph, 205
　scientific developments leading to, 202-208
　treatment addiction using, 213-214

## O

Obesity, 182-186
　as a metabolic disorder, 183
　complications of, 183
　current emphasis on dietary fat and cholesterol, 186
　diet of Japan, 185
　difficulty treating, 183-184
　exercise to maintain or lose weight, 183, 220
　formation trans-fatty acids, 186
　incidence people on reducing schemes, 183
　"mood foods," 184
　overrated belief, 182
　pear-shaped women, 182-183
　popular diet schemes, 184-185
　proper diet, 219-220
　role of physician in treatment of, 183
　treatment as a lucrative business, 184
　upper body fat, 182
　"yo-yo" effect, 183
Office of Alternative Medicine, National Institutes of Health, xiii, 16
Orgone therapy, 147
O-ring test, 5, 111-112
Orthomolecular medicine, 191
Osteopathic medicine, 137-140
　definition, 138
　examination and treatment, 139-140
　founding of, 137-138
　medications used, 140
　nature of, 138-139
　　manipulation used, 138-139
　　wholistic medicine practiced, 138
　number licensed today, 138
　origin of term, 137
　summary, 140
Out of body experience (OBE), 32

## P

Pain, 208-214, 220
　acupuncture for control of, 211-212 (*see also* Electro-acupuncture)
　analgesia from body manipulations, 210
　and the nervous system, 209-210
　biofeedback (*see* Biofeedback)

chiropractic (*see* Chiropractic medicine)
gate theory, 203
induction analgesia, 210
  by opioid peptides, 210
  by serotonin, 210
jogger's high, 210
methods of controlling, 210-211
nature of, 208-209
need for, 208
neuroelectric acupuncture (*see* Neuroelectric acupuncture)
osteopathy (*see* Osteopathy medicine)
pain behavior, 208
phantom limb pain, 211
regulation of, 209-210
studies chemicals in brain for control of, 204
  results of, graph, 204
types of, 208-209
use electro-acupuncture to decrease, 210 (*see also* Electro-acupuncture)
use of "pain pills," 211
Palmistry, 112-113
  typical beliefs of, 113
Parapsychology, 31-33
astral projections, 32
beginning of, 31
clairvoyance and precognition, 31
extrasensory perception, 31-32
first studies of, 32
near death experience, 32
out of body experience, 32
precognition, 31, 34
*psi* phenomena studies, 33
psychokinesis, 31, 33
reincarnation, 32
telepathy, 31
unidentified flying objects, 32
use of term, 31
Peptic ulcer
allopathic treatment, 152
alternative treatment, 152
Phantom limb pain, control of, 211
Physical health
education, 73
effect religious commitment on, 72-73
metastatic breast cancer, 73-74
relationship blood pressure and, 73
smoking, 73
Placebo medicine, 50-56, 159
blockage effect of, 55
conclusions, 56
conditions responding to, 53
current use of, 53-54
double-blind studies, 52
effect doctor-patient relationship, 54
effect of, 53
impeding heading, 51
importance of, 54
mechanism of, 54-55
  relief of anxiety, 54-55
medical practices forming placebos, 51
neuropeptide hypothesis, 55
new drugs as not effective for everybody, 51
  role of placebo in, 51-52
  use double-blind experiments, 52
patient demand for pills, 56

placebo effect, xviii, 14-15
positive thinking and, 56
production of miracles, 51
Random Clinical Trial (RCT), 52
responses to explained, 55
role in treatments used by healers, 54
side-effects produced by, 53
study of angina pectoris and, 53
study personality responders to, 55
summary, 220-221
total drug effect formula, 52
use in evaluating new drugs' effectiveness, 50-51
use of herbology, 51
Polarity therapy, 144
Precognition, 31, 34
Progressive relaxation, 80
Prostate enlargement
allopathic treatment, 151
alternative treatment, 151
Pseudomedicine
Ayurvedic medicine as, 104
caution of printed articles, 102
essentials for selling, 100-101
*meridian* theory myth of acupuncture, 103
mindset basic to, 100
New Age products selling tactics, 101-102
role greed in, 102
truisms used in selling, 101-102
*Psi* phenomena, 32-33 (*see also* Spiritualism)
Psionic diagnosis, 113-114
Psychokinesis
definition, 31
by Uri Geller, 33
Psychological distress, effect religious states on, 72
Psychology, origin of term, 69
Psychosomatic medicine
definition, 6
illnesses cited as, 10
teaching of in U.S. medical schools, 46

## Q

*Qi Gong*, 4-5, 17, 40
energy occurring due to, 40
feedback therapy, 5, 17
in U.S., 5
investigation of, 5
O-Ring technique, 5, 111-112
practice of in China, 21-22
types of, 4
use relaxation in, 79 (*see also* Relaxation)
*Qi Gong*-feedback-therapy (QFT), 5, 17
Quackery
definition, 98
source of term, 98, 157

## R

Radiesthesia, 113-114
dowsing, 113
Radionics, 113-114
Random Clinical Trial (RCT), use of, 52
Reflexology, 144
Reiki healing, 38, 81, 144-145, 146-147
Reincarnation, 32
Relaxation, 79-94
autogenic training system, 80

biofeedback, 81-86 (*see also* Biofeedback)
homeostasis (*see* Homeostasis)
hypnosis, 87-94 (*see also* Hypnosis)
   in Ayurvedic medicine, 79
   in holistic treatments, 79
   interaction sympathetic and parasympathetic systems, 79-80
   progressive, 80
   relaxation response, 80-81
   response of Benson, 80-81
   techniques using, 81
   use isolation tanks, 81
   use visual imagery, 81
Religious healings, 5-6
Rolfing massage technique, 143-144
Rosecrucian healing, 38

**S**

Scalp acupuncture, 146
Seance, definition, 29
"Seat of the soul," 44
Shamanism (*see also* Magical healing)
   bio-psycho-social-spiritual healing, 27
   changes induced by, 28
   contemporary, 27
      Edgar Cayce, 27-28
   cultural factors in, 28
   definition, 4
   description, 4
   Early Oriental healing, 4
   faith in as healer, 74
   healing of, 25, 27
   mysterious behavior of, 28
   *Qi Gong*, 4- 5

   responsibilities of, 25
   source of term, 24
   unscientific methods of diagnosis, 106
   use of medicine man by American Indians, 25-27
   use of today, 24
Sinarteriology
   basis of, 122
   definition, 122
Society for Psychical Research, founding of, 31
Somatic biofeedback, 84
Sonopuncture, 146
Southampton Diet, 184-185
Spiritualism, 29-31
   beginning of movement, 29
   definitions, 29
   exposure by Houdini, 30
   mediums, 29
   seance, 29
   spread of movement, 30-31
Suicide, lower rates religious persons, 71

**T**

T'ai Chi C'huan, 145-146
Tarot fortune telling, 35
Telepathy, definition, 31
Therapeutic massage, 143
   techniques of, 143-144
Therapeutic Touch, 38, 144-145
   energy from, 41-42
Thermal biofeedback, 83
Thoughts, 45
Traditional Chinese acupuncture, 196-215 (*see also* Acupuncture)
Trager massage technique, 144
Traditional Chinese Medicine

acupuncture (*see* Acupuncture)
concept of illness, 199
concepts of *Yin* and *Yang*, 39, 40-41, 123, 199
    pairs of, table, 124
    waxing and waning of, illustration, 124
evolutive phases of, 123, 125, 127
    diagram of, 126
five element theory, 199
    diagram, 200, 201
    evolutive (productive) phase, 199-200
forms of energy, 128
herbology, 11-13, 128 (*see also* Herbology and homeopathy)
holistic treatment, 127
Law of Wu Hing, 200-201
    *Ko* cycle, 200, 201
    *Sheng* cycle, 200, 201
    table of, 201
*meridians* theory, 8, 103, 108, 122, 197
    traditional, table, 1 98
    unpaired, table, 198
preventive medicine, 128
pulses used for diagnosis, 127, 200
    location of, illustration, 108-109, 126, 200
scientization of, 17
surgeries included in, 128
treatments of, 200 C.E. and today, 128
unscientific diagnostic methods in, 108-110
    basic concept, 108
    pulse diagnosis, 108-109
    use of *meridians*, 108
    use of general anesthesia, 128
    use relaxation in, 79 (*see also* Relaxation)
Transcendental meditation concept, 120

## U

Unconventional medicine comprehensive systems, 116-152
    Ayurvedic Medicine (*see* Ayurvedic Medicine)
    chiropractic medicine (*see* Chiropractic medicine)
    osteopathy medicine (*see* Osteopathy medicine)
    sideshows of alternative medicine, 140-147 (*see also* Alternative medicine)
    Traditional Chinese Medicine (*see* Traditional Chinese Medicine)
    treatments-allopathic and alternative, 147-152
        anxiety-insomnia, 148
        arthritis, 148
        asthma-hay fever, 149
        common cold, 150
        diabetes, 150
        focus of each, 147
        headache, 151
        hypertension, 149
        peptic ulcer, 152
        prostate enlargement, 151
Unidentified flying objects, 32

## V

Vibrational healing, 146
Vitamins and minerals, 189-191
    cautions in purchase of, 189
    dose schedule of, table, 191
    megavitamin therapy, 191
    RDA listings of, 189
    reputed beneficial effects
        vitamin supplementation, 190-191
    supplementation of, 189, 190
        added to food products, 190
    vitamin combinations used for arthritis, 191
    vitamin uses suggested, 190
        table, 194-195
    vitamins defined, 189
    vitamins stored in body, 190
        excess of, 190

Voodoo of Africa healing, 4

## W

Wu, of China, 4

## Y

*Yin* and *Yang*
    balance of for wellness, 40-41
    concepts of, 123, 199
    meaning of terms, 39
    pairs of, table, 124
    waxing and waning of, illustration, 124

*Yoga*
    associated with Ayurveda, 119
    emphasis on energy sources, 120
        illustration, 121
    methods used in U.S., 119
    types exercises, 119-120